FUNCTIONAL REHABILITATION of SOME COMMON NEUROLOGICAL CONDITIONS

FUNCTIONAL REHABILITATION of SOME COMMON NEUROLOGICAL CONDITIONS

A Physical Management Strategy to Optimise
Functional Activity Level

Sayeed Ahmed MCSP.

Copyright © 2019 by Sayeed Ahmed MCSP..

ISBN: Softcover   978-1-5434-9446-4
             eBook   978-1-5434-9445-7

All rights reserved. No part of this book may be reproduced or transmitted in any form or by any means, electronic or mechanical, including photocopying, recording, or by any information storage and retrieval system, without permission in writing from the copyright owner.

This is a work of fiction. Names, characters, places and incidents either are the product of the author's imagination or are used fictitiously, and any resemblance to any actual persons, living or dead, events, or locales is entirely coincidental.

Any people depicted in stock imagery provided by Getty Images are models, and such images are being used for illustrative purposes only.
Certain stock imagery © Getty Images.

Print information available on the last page.

Rev. date: 02/27/2019

To order additional copies of this book, contact:
Xlibris
800-056-3182
www.Xlibrispublishing.co.uk
Orders@Xlibrispublishing.co.uk
790585

CONTENTS

PHYSICAL MANAGEMENT STRATEGY TO RESTORE SENSORY-MOTOR FUNCTION AND TO REGAIN FUNCTIONAL AUTONOMY IN PEOPLE WITH POST STROKE HEMIPLEGIA

I: Introduction 3
II: Restoration of Neural Function Following a Stroke 8
 - Experience-dependent change in the brain tissues..............9
 - Functional reorganisation in the intact neural circuits 11
 - Lesion induced cell proliferative activity 12
III: Functional Architecture of the Nervous System that Mediates Motor Activities 19
 - Program control system of the brain................................22
 - Feedback control system of the brain..............................26
 - Reflex control system..29
IV: Consequence of Stroke on the Motor Controlling System of the Brain 38
 - Impaired programme control system of the brain 39
 - Impaired feedback control system of the brain................39
 - Uninhibited and non-modulated reflex muscle activities......42
V: Strategy to Restore Impaired Structure of Functional Architecture Central Nervous System that Mediates Kinematic Motor Organisation 55
 - Activities to restore feedback controlled system in the brain..56
 - Activities to restore program control system in the brain......62
 - The physical management of uninhibited reflex activities or spasticity...80
VI: Restore Sensory Function 84
VII: Restore Balance Function in People Following a Stroke.........90

VIII:	Different Cognitive Dysfunctions in Hemiplegic Subjects and their Repercussion in Attaining Functional Recovery	101
IX:	Strategies to Minimise the Difficulty to Relearning Muscle Function in People with Attention Dysfunction	130
X:	Conclusion	149

A GUIDE TO UPHOLD PHYSICAL ACTIVITY LEVEL IN PEOPLE WITH PARKINSON'S DISEASE

I:	Introduction	169
II:	A Brief Anatomy Physiology of Basal Ganglia and Some Associated Motor Areas	175
	- The nuclei of basal ganglia	176
	- Connections of basal ganglia	176
	- Connection of basal ganglia within themselves	177
	- Connection of basal ganglia and other areas of brain	177
III:	Function of Basal Ganglia	179
	- Function of basal ganglia as storing and retrieving structure of motor activities	180
	- The role of neurotransmitter for the proper functioning of the basal ganglia and their connection and some underlying factors responsible for the Parkinson disease symptoms	181
	- Role of different motor areas in generating movements	183
IV:	Diagnosis of Parkinson's Disease	186
V:	Early Dementia	188
VI:	Fall and Instability in PD	189
VII:	The Repercussion of Defective Dopamine Metabolism on the Functional Architecture of the Nervous System that Mediates Motor Activities	190
	- Possible movement strategies to ease difficulty to perform the three functional tasks at home	211
VIII:	Strategies to Minimise Walking and Turning Difficulties in PD Subject	229
IX:	Cognitive Impairments in PD Subjects and their Repercussion on Functional Activity Level	248

X: Possibility to Foster Neural Changes in Parkinson Subjects in Order to Assure Long Term Functional Improvement...262

REHABILITATION OF PEOPLE WITH TRAUMATIC PARAPLEGIA

I: Introduction...285
II: Management in the Acute Stage, During Bed Rest Period...286
III: Treatment in the Chronic Stage When Bed Rest is Over.....289
- Progressive standing practice 289
- Improve sitting balance 289
- Strengthening of the upper limb and trunk muscles 290
- Learn to use wheel chair in daily life activities 290
- Reintegration into social, professional life and participate sportive activities..290

PHYSICAL MANAGEMENT GUIDE FOR PEOPLE WITH MULTIPLE SCLEROSIS

I: Introduction...295
II: Physiopathology of MS..297
III: Physical Management of Motor Impairment in Multiple Sclerosis 299
- Restore balance function 299
- Restoration of program control system 303
- Restore feedback control system 303
- Management of spasticity.......................................304
IV: Improve Functional Activities Level and Engaging in an Aerobic Activity..305
V: Cognitive Impairment and Possibility to Facilitate Neural Changes in Multiple Sclerosis 307
VI: Conclusion..309

PHYSICAL MANAGEMENT STRATEGY TO RESTORE SENSORY-MOTOR FUNCTION AND TO REGAIN FUNCTIONAL AUTONOMY IN PEOPLE WITH POST STROKE HEMIPLEGIA

1
Introduction

Human motor skills, which produce dynamic activities in order to achieve different functional goals, are the result of an organised kinematic activity of different muscles. Hochstenbach and Mulder (1999) have stated that the motor skills have a specific organisational structure and the components of movement patterns are interrelated and dependent on each other. Moreover the study of brain's functional architecture unveils that this organised activity of multiple muscles (kinematic motor organisation) during different functional tasks, is mediated by three distinct functional systems within the central nervous system. They are program control system, feedback control system, and reflex control systems. The program control system retrieves previously learned muscle activities, which consist of a chain of interrelated and mutually dependent muscle action; the feedback control system provides the strength and dexterity of individual muscle into this retrieved muscle chain for the successful accomplishment of kinematic motor organisation; and reflex control system helps to shape the kinematic motor organisation by providing inhibited and modulated reflex muscle activities. In addition, this organised structure is specific for each task. What is more, that these organised activities are not the result of only muscle function but different sensory and cognitive functions also contribute in this organisation process. A breakdown of the kinematic motor organisation occurs in a cerebro-vascular-accident (CVA). In particular, the damage of feedback and program control system is responsible for the beak down of this organisational structure. Moreover the unimpaired reflex control system is left alone to function. Not only the intact reflex control system continues to generate the reflex muscle activities following a CVA, but also they are deprived of their inhibiting and modulation effect from the two other systems and become the predominant muscle activities aftermath of a CVA. Given that different sensory and cognitive functions play an important role in the generation of kinematic motor organisation, the impaired cognitive and sensory functions can aggravate the severity of the functional impairment following a CVA. A neuronal damage within the brain is the underlying cause of these impairments; and the restoration of neuronal function is therefore crucial to re-establish the brain's ability to generate organised motor activities. In contrast a failure to restore neural function can perpetuate the impaired of brain function, and the deficit of generation of interrelated, interdependent, and organised motor activities may remain prevalent. The restoration of neural function up to a certain extent is possible, because human brain is endowed with neurogenesis activities. This restoration again is depended on the extent of neural damage; and the appropriate stimulations received by the brain following a brain damage. New brain imaging techniques are making it clear that the neural system is continually remodelled throughout the life and after injury by experience and learning in response to activity and behaviour (Jenkins et al 1990, Johnsson 2000, Nudo et al 2001). In both humans and animals, data shows that in the hippocampus, new cells can indeed be produced (Eriksson et al 1989, Gould et al 1999). Seitz (1995) states that plastic changes occur in the damaged brain and Robertson (1999) suggest that these changes mediate in part recovery of function after brain damage. Moreover Kokotilo et al (2010) states that the functional reorganisation of the central nervous system is thought to be one of the fundamental mechanisms involved in recovery of neurological injury, such as stroke. The mechanism of change in the brain following a stroke includes; - an experience-dependent or stimulation-dependent change in the brain tissues; - a functional reorganisation in the intact neural circuits; and - a lesion induced neuronal proliferative activity. Different stimulations in form of activity and behaviour can facilitate the above changes in the damaged brain in people with stroke. Those neural changes can eventually maximise the recovery of brain function, which in turn can help to regain its capacity to generate kinematic organisation of motor activities. However precisely what kind of experience to provide in order to facilitate recovery is problematic: non-specific stimulation can inadvertently strengthen non-damaged competitor circuits, or it might simply fail to provide the type of precisely shaped and timed input that is needed to foster changes in a particular lesioned network (Robertson 1999). This problem can be minimised by elucidating brain's functional architecture. It can in turn help to identify the parts of the functional architecture that are damaged and the parts that are not damaged. This knowledge in turn can be the guide for providing the appropriate therapeutic stimulations that are needed to restore impaired neural function. Moreover elucidating the brain's functional architecture can make contribution towards the development of a scientific basis for the practice of brain rehabilitation. The data generated from the rehabilitation-oriented research can be tested to identify the stimulations that are effective to restore the structure of functional architecture of the nervous system that are damaged. According to Robertson (1999) rehabilitation – the provision of planned experience to foster brain changes leading to improved daily life functioning – can now therefore turn its sights to the ambitious goal of directly altering neural circuitry through appropriately planned experience. Given that program and feedback control systems are impaired in a CVA, therefore the precisely shaped stimulations following a stroke are those which can restore these two systems of the brain.

As the neural recovery is the most essential factor in the restoring process of functional recovery following a stroke; therefore the first chapter describes the mechanism of neural changes that can be fostered, which includes neural changes in an intact as well as in a damaged brain. Different type neural changes, like experience-dependent change of brain tissues, functional reorganisation in the intact neural circuits, and lesion induced cell proliferative activities that take place in a brain, are discussed. Then the possibility of facilitate these changes in stroke is also examined. The factors that facilitate neural changes and the factors that have interfering effect on the neutral change are also discussed.

In chapter on the role of brain in generating muscle activities investigates the functional architecture of the brain that mediates kinematic motor organisation. The discussion integrates clinical research findings that explain the three distinct systems of the brain that are responsible for this organisation process. Mak and Cole (1991) have elaborated on two distinct systems of the brain in mediating muscle activities. These systems include program control system, feedback control system. Moreover a third system which plays a role in kinematic organisation of muscle activities is reflex muscle activities. The program controlled system is largely responsible for the kinematic motor organisation of learned movements. The feedback controlled system produces individual muscle action, where conscious and voluntary efforts play an important role in generating muscle activities. The reflex muscle activities generate different reflex and postural activities of muscle. The understanding of these three systems, which belongs to brain's functional architectural entity is essential in providing precisely shaped stimulation to facilitate the restoration of impaired brain function and avoid inadvertently strength the non damaged competitor circuits.

Both the feedback controlled and program controlled activities can be affected following a brain stroke; whereas the reflex controlled activities often remain intact after a stroke. Moreover in a normal circumstance the feedback and program controlled activities exert modulating and inhibiting effects on different reflex controlled activities, and impairment of these two systems may eliminate these effects. Consequently reflex activities become a dominant muscle activity following a stroke. Therefore the consequences of stroke on different muscle controlling system is described, which in turn can provide us with better understanding regarding different appropriate stimulations that are needed to facilitate neural change.

Given that the muscle dysfunction after a stroke results from an impaired feedback control and program control system of the brain, therefore the rehabilitation strategies have tried to expose the precisely shaped stimulations that facilitate the restoration of these two systems in the brain. The chapter on restoration of impaired brain function has integrated clinical research finding to provide a guideline of exercise program that constitute the precisely shaped stimulation for restoring these two systems. Not only research based evidences but also the knowledge of neuropsychological function is used to identify the precisely shaped stimulation that can help to restore impaired brain function. Improving individual muscle function is essential to restore feedback control system, which can be achieved by improving strength and dexterity of individual muscle. Therefore the possible strategies to improve individual muscle function in reflex inhibition position are also discussed. Whereas in the process of restoration of program control system different functional exercise and whole muscle chain exercises constitute precisely shaped stimulation.

Certain cognitive functions play an essential role in the mediation of kinematic organisation of motor activities during functional tasks. Different cognitive functions are also crucial in the relearning of motor function and reacquisition of functional autonomy. Moreover experience-dependent plastic reorganisation depends on attention being paid by the recipient to the stimulation responsible for such. In other words people with impaired cognitive function may not be able attend to the provided stimulation, which may not be able to facilitate change in the damaged brain. Therefore the chapter on cognitive function has discussed some common cognitive impairment in stroke, their interaction on the restoration of impaired brain function, and finally the impact of different cognitive dysfunctions on re-learning of motor function and reacquisition of functional autonomy.

The last chapter has examined the secondary impairments of musculo-skeletal structures in hemiplegic subjects. After a stroke, inactivity of the limb can produce a wide range of function and structural changes in muscles, bones, tendons and ligaments. These changes are mainly due to stress deprivation of tissues, and changes of musculo-skeletal structures can further aggravate functional disability. The underlying mechanisms of these changes and then possibility to minimise these changes are also examined.

II

Restoration of Neural Function Following a Stroke

Introduction: Muscle dysfunction leading to a functional incapacity in people aftermath of a stroke is linked to the neuronal damage within the brain. Therefore the objective of rehabilitation strategy is to restore neural function. The restoration of neural function to a certain extent is possible, depending on the extent of damage and the appropriateness of the rehabilitation strategy. Fostering of changes like 'experience-dependent change' (Recanzone et al 1993) and 'functional reorganisation' (Luria 1975) within the intact neural circuit of a damaged brain and facilitation of neuronal proliferation activities are possible following a brain damage. These types of neuronal changes contribute largely the functional recovery of post-stroke hemiplegic subjects. Bach-y-Rita P (1989) suggests that certain circumstances rehabilitation might even have direct neural effects. Recent neuroimaging studies in humans have demonstrated that reorganisation of brain activation relates to functional outcome after stroke (Dong et al 2007, Dong et al 2006, Ward et al 2003). According to Luria (1975) rehabilitation following brain damage has its effect by fostering 'functional reorganisation'- the compensatory reorganisation of surviving undamaged brain in order to achieve impaired behaviour goal in different way. Moreover Robertson (1999) suggests that such mechanisms do indeed underpin much behavioural recovery. Another theory proposed by Robertson (1999) which is that the recovery from brain damage may take to be a result of the activity of healthy circuits working to remove inhibitors from the damaged networks. This can take place either by dampening down the inhibitory competition, or by boosting the activation in circuits in the lesioned network. Robertson (1999) has therefore concluded that it is likely that many if not all of these mechanisms are important in the recovery from brain damage – whether such recovery is spontaneous, or guided by a structured program known as rehabilitation. Yet the question as to precisely what kind of experience to provide in order to facilitate recovery is itself highly problematic, since any non-specific stimulation might inadvertently strengthen non damaged competitor circuits while failing to provide the type of precisely shaped and timed input needed to foster changes in a particular lesioned network.

Robertson (1999) goes on to claim that rehabilitation – the provision of planned experience to foster brain changes leading to improved daily life functioning – can now therefore turn its sights to the ambitious goal of directly altering neural circuitry through appropriate planned experience. It is in this context the following discussion will examine the literature on experience-dependent change', 'lesion induced change' and 'functional reorganisation', as well as examining the possibility of promoting these changes in people following a stroke.

- Experience dependent change in the brain tissue.
- Functional reorganisation in the intact neural circuits
- Lesion induced neuron proliferative activities.

Experience-dependent change in the brain tissues:

Research carried out by Eriksson et al (1998) and Gould et al (1999) suggests that new cells are produced in the hippocampus of the adult human brain. Similarly Gould et al (1997), Kempermann, et al (1997) and Cameron (1993) have demonstrated from stereological analyses that several thousand hipocamppal cells produced each day in adult animals, the majority of which differentiate into granulate neurones. Moreover Gould et al (1999) suggest that if granule neurons produced in adulthood is necessary for hipocampal function in certain types of learning and memory, then regulatory factors that diminish the production of new neurons should be associated with impaired learning while those that enhance the production of new neurones should improve learning.

Moreover these changes are experience-dependent; animals kept in enriched compared to impoverished show more cell genesis in the hippocampus (Kempermann et al 1998). They have demonstrated that more hippocampal granule neurons are sustained in mice living in an 'enriched environment' as compared to conditions in a laboratory cage. Praag.et al (1999), examined the impact of running, and Gould et al (1999), whose work was concerned with specific learning tasks, have demonstrated the impact of such activity in promoting neurogenesis and neural survival in the adult mouse hippocampus. The latter, however, admits that that the extent to which this increase in the number of surviving granule cells following environmental enrichment may directly contribute to an improved hippocampal function remains unknown. This notwithstanding, it is clear that the brain responds to external stimulation in the form of different activities by producing more neurons and axonal connections. In contrast the absence of such stimulation may well explain its failure to undertake this process of cell genesis.

Elbert et al (1995) observed that right-handed string players show an increased cortical representation (map) of flexor and extensor muscles for the fingers of the left but not the right hand. Moreover it is observed that the sensori-motor cortical representation of the reading finger is expanded in blind Braille readers (Pascal-Leone and Torres 1993) and fluctuates according to the extent of reading activities (Pascal-Leone et al 1995). These types of cortical representations (map) remain enlarged with regular practice (Elbart et al 1995). In contrast restriction activity may decrease cortical representation of different muscles. Liepert et al (1995) have demonstrated a significant decrease in the cortical motor representation of inactive leg muscles after 4-6 weeks of unilateral ankle immobilisation and was more pronounced when the duration of immobilisation was longer. Therefore it is clear that in human new neurons including axonal and dendritic sprouting can take place. However this process is partly experience-dependent or stimulation-dependent; that is, neurogenasis can be facilitated in people who receive stimulation and this process can be absent in people who are deprived of stimulation.

Moreover there is emerging evidence in animal models that pharmacotherapy, learning, and exercise may have a neuroprotective influence in neurological disorders. Woodlee and Schallert (2004) found that the onset of abnormal movements to be prevented or delayed when parkinsonien rats exposed to MPTP (1-methyl-4-phenyl-1,2,3,6-tetrahydropyridine) were trained in an enriched environment. Similarly rat models on Huntington disease have shown that locomotors training using a treadmill delays the progression of gait disorders (Spires and Hannan 2005). Therefore different appropriate exercise programmes as part of rehabilitation not only enhances experience-dependent change but also prevent development of abnormal movement pattern in people after stroke.

Functional reorganisation in the intact neural circuits:

An appropriate stimulation may be responsible for the expansion movement representation in the intact areas of the brain. The territories that were speared after stroke may be progressively atrophied and could eventually lack its representation capacity in case of stimulation deprivation. In contrast repeated stimulation to achieved impaired movement may facilitate a 'functional reorganisation' in the intact neural circuits- the compensatory reorganisation of unaffected brain circuits in order to achieve the impaired functional goals in a different way (Lauria 1963; Lauria et al 1975) and thus help to facilitate functional recovery. According to Carr and Shepherd (2004) studies on animals and humans with brain lesions provide insight into the process of functional recovery, which reflect the relationship between the neural reorganisation and rehabilitation process.

Modern cortical mapping techniques in both non-human and human subject indicate that the functional organisation of the primary motor cortex is much more complex than was traditionally described (Carr and Shepherd 2004). The complex organisation has extensive overlapping of muscle representation within the motor map, with individual muscle and joint representations re-represented within the motor map, individual corticospinal neurons diverging to multiple motoneuron pools, and horizontal fibres interconnecting distributed representations and this complex organisation may provide the foundation for functional plasticity in the motor cortex (Nudo et al 2001).

Experiment by Nudo et al (1996) demonstrated that following a lesion to a small part of the motor cortex of the squirrel monkey, hand-movement representations adjacent to the area of the infract that were spared from direct injury underwent further loss of cortical territory. However an intensive training of skilled hand use resulted in a prevention of the loss of hand territory adjacent to the infarct area. In some instances, they found that the hand representations expanded into region formerly occupied by representations of the shoulder and elbow. The brain tissue loss could have been due to non-use of the hand and this was confirmed by a follow-up study which showed that not only could tissue loss be prevented, when unimpaired hand was restrained and the monkey had daily repetitive training in skilled use of the impaired hand, but there was also a net gain of approximately 10% in the total hand area adjacent to the lesion (Nudo et al 1996). Another study by Friel and Nudo (1989), in which the unimpaired hand was restrained but no training was given, the size of the total hand representation decreased, indicating that restrain of the unimpaired hand alone was not sufficient to retain the spread hand area. The results of these studies point to the necessity for active use of the limb for the survival of undamaged neurons adjacent to those damaged by cortical injury, and suggest that retention of the spread of the hand area and recovery of function after cortical injury might depend upon repetitive training and skilled use of hand (Nudo and Friel 1999).The authors concluded that rehabilitative training can shape subsequent reorganisation in the intact cortex. However it has been noted that soon after stroke the excitability of the motor cortex is decreased and the cortical representations are reduced (Carr and Shepherd 2004). Therefore the repeated stimulation can not only prevent the expansion of neuronal atrophy but also facilitate the establishment of cortical representation by the intact neural circuits.

Neuron proliferation after brain lesion:

Evidence suggests that the cell proliferative activities are enhanced following a brain lesion. For example study conducted by Cao et al

(2002) has demonstrated that lesion-induced cell loss facilitate cell proliferative activities; that is the loss of cells in one area of the brain facilitate cell proliferation on the other areas, possibly to facilitate the compensation of functional losses. Cao et al (2002) conclude from their research that adult brain of mammals and birds are not generally endowed with mechanisms of cell repair. They however, suggest that lesion and/or lesion-induced cell loss facilitate cell proliferative activity in subventricular zone, concurrently induced morphological changes which may provide a favourable environment for local neuron recruitment. Similarly research carried out by Recanzone et al (1993) has demonstrated that following brain damage, the adult brain can show large experience-dependent change in the intact neural circuits, including dendritic and axonal sprouting. According to Robertson (1999) such changes mediate in part recovery of function after brain damage. It is clear then that after stroke there is increased cell proliferative activity in the intact neural circuits to compensate functional loss of the brain. However the retention and maturation of proliferated neurons largely depend on the stimulation received by the subjects; and a no challenging environment or stimulation deprivation may lead to disintegration of newly proliferated neurones. An appropriate and timely rehabilitation program is therefore essential to facilitate retention and maturation of lesion induced proliferated neurons.

Possible appropriate rehabilitation to facilitate neural change following a stroke:

Little is known about the parameters such as timing, duration, and the frequency of different stimulations to obtain this type of experience-dependent change (Robertson 1999). One aspect is clear that experience-dependent change and functional reorganisation after a CVA is facilitated when the task is active dynamic and repeated. Moreover cell proliferative activities occur after stroke and retention and maturation of newly proliferative cells depends on the stimulation received by the newly proliferated neurons. Neural reorganisation occurs in the human cortex after stroke and altered neural activity patterns and molecular events influence this functional reorganisation which is demonstrated by Johansson (2000) who carried out neuroimaging and non-invasive stimulation studies – positron emission tomography (PET), functional magnetic resonance imaging (fMIRI) and transcranial magnetic stimulation (TMS), these investigations have also demonstrated that the cerebral cortex is functionally and structurally dynamic. One theory put forward by Carre and Shepherd (2004) in relation to people after stroke, proposes that the changes in the brain cells associated with skill development can be provoked by active, repetitive training and practice, and by the continued practice of the activity. Conversely inactivity may deprive the brain the necessary stimulation for facilitating neural change necessary for functional recovery. That is a non-challenging environment may hinder this process of experience dependent change in the brain.

The proliferation and retention of brain cells as well as their axonal and dendritic sporting are experience-dependent. That is the cell proliferation as well as their axonal and dendritic sprouting is enhanced in human and in animal living in an enriched environment compared to those who are living in a deprived environment. Different stimulations in form of experience and learning may foster neural changes. Therefore an appropriate exercise programme provides precisely shaped experience to facilitate neural recovery in people after stroke. Appropriate stimulations are those which can provide stimulation to the impaired neural networks and eventually facilitate their restoration. An appropriate exercise programme not only facilitates neural recovery but also prevents their further atrophy and then development of abnormal movements. However different cognitive impairments can have hindering effect on the process of neural change. The process of experience-dependent change is hindered in people with impaired attention function. In addition, increase in synaptic efficacy in the existing neural circuits in the form of long-term potentiation and formation of new synapses may be involved in earlier stages of motor learning (Asanuma and Keller1991). The principal process responsible for functional recovery beyond the immediate reparative stage is likely be use-dependent reorganisation of the neural mechanism (Carre and Shepherd 2004). They further suggest that adaptive plasticity is inevitable after an acute brain lesion, and it is very likely that rehabilitation may influence it. A systemic review carried out by Kokotilo et al (2009) of 26 studies on forced production in stroke showed that persons with stroke are more likely to activate motor areas when using their paretic limb, such as the ipsilesional primary motor cortex, premotor cortex, supplementary motor areas, parietal cortex, and cerebellum. It seems essential that that rehabilitation program include active and repetitive practice, that it tries to restore impaired functional losses of the brain, and that the program is adapted taking in to account of different cognitive impairments.

Cognitive function and neural change:

Cognitive function plays an important role in facilitating neural change. It is an important aspect for consideration because stroke can result in an impaired cognitive function. According to Robertson et al (1997) the attentional systems of the brain might have a privileged role in the recovery of function after brain damage. The process of experience-dependent change may be hindered in subjects with impaired attention function. Not only attention dysfunction but also other cognitive dysfunctions like impaired executive function or memory dysfunction may have hindering effect on the retention of newly proliferated brain cells as well as development of axonal and dedritic sprouting. Lewis et al (2003) have demonstrated that human models with impaired executive function there are specific under-activity in the striatum as well as in the frontal cortex during performance of working-memory task compare to group with no significant executive impairments. Therefore people with cognitive dysfunction will have poor functional recovery, compare to those without significant cognitive dysfunction. In other word people with impaired cognitive function may not be benefited from the stimulations provided in form of therapeutic activities; as if they are living in a deprived environment. People with cognitive dysfunction are often dependent on other people for the activities of daily living; this passive living condition can be responsible for the stimulation deprivation for the injured brain, which in turn may have hindering effect on neural changes. However it might be possible to minimise the negative influence of impaired cognitive function, that is the rehabilitation strategy has to be adapted taking in to account the presence of cognitive impairment. More detailed description on possible adaptive strategy in case of cognitive dysfunction is cited in the chapter on cognitive function. It is evident that cognitive impairment is responsible for poor prognosis after stroke, however the negative influence of cognitive dysfunction may be minimise if the rehabilitation strategies can be adapted according to cognitive dysfunctions.

In addition, in order to facilitate neurogensis, an environment for learning motor skills and functional activities is indispensable for the stroke patients. Stress or aging which are associated with elevated adrenaline can suppress neurogenesis. Kuhn et al (1996) demonstrate that the stress or aging are accompanied by diminished granule cell production in both rodents and primates. Therefore, it is important to ensure that the learning environment does not create extra stress for the patients.

Conclusion: Human brain is endowed with a wide range of neural changes. These changes include experience-dependent change and functional reorganisation. Moreover following a brain damage there can be cell proliferative activities in the brain.

In experience-dependent change there is formation of new neurons as well as dendritic and axonal sprouting within the brain tissue. Different experiences like education and exercise provide stimulation to the brain to facilitate cell genesis in the brain, whereas stimulation deprivation may hinder this process.

There may also be functional reorganisation in the damaged brain – 'the compensatory reorganisation of surviving undamaged brain circuit in order to achieve the impaired behavioural goal in a different way' (Lauria et al 1975). An appropriate stimulation can facilitate functional reorganisation. In contrast stimulation deprivation may not only fail to facilitate functional reorganisation, but also enhance the propagation neural atrophy beyond the damaged area of the brain.

Moreover brain lesion like stroke boosts cell proliferative activities within the brain, probably to compensate functional loss of the brain. However retention and maturation of newly proliferated neurons depends on the stimulation provided.

It may be assumed that experience-dependent change and functional reorganisation can be facilitated in the brain after stroke, and that such changes mediate in part recovery of function in people after stroke. However the most experiments on neural changes are done either on animals or on healthy human being. Moreover cognitive dysfunctions can have a hindering effect in the process of neural change. Many stroke patients are elderly and often their brain may be affected by degenerative changes even before their stroke and they can have different degrees of cognitive dysfunctions, which can have hindering effect on the neural change. In addition inappropriate stimulation may stimulate competitor circuits and may have hindering effect on functional recovery. Therefore more research is needed to identify the appropriate stimulation that can facilitate neural changes and assure functional recovery after stroke.

Summary of the restoration of neural function after a stroke:

- The human brain is endowed with changes, which include proliferation new neurons as well as dendritic and axonal sprouting.
- Three types of neuron proliferative activities can take place in brain following a stroke; they are: - experience dependent change; - functional reorganisation and ; - lesion induced neuron proliferative activities
- In experience-dependent change different stimulations in form of exercises and experiences facilitate new neuron production as well as dendritic and axonal sprouting, whereas stimulation deprivation may hinder these changes.
- Different active exercises after a brain damage may facilitate functional reorganisation– 'the compensatory reorganisation of surviving undamaged brain circuit in order to achieve the impaired behavioural goal in a different way' (Lauria et al 1975). In contrast stimulation deprivation may be responsible for the propagation neural atrophy beyond the damaged area of the brain.

- Following a brain lesion like stroke there may enhance neuronal proliferative activities within the brain, probably to compensate functional loss of the brain.
- Retention and maturation of newly proliferated neurons depend on the stimulation received by the hemiplegic subjects.
- Functional recovery after stroke is largely depended on the possibility to facilitate the above neuronal changes.
- Repeated exercise of the whole muscle chain and functional exercises seem to be appropriate stimulation since they use the inter related and interdependent muscle chain.
- In contrast inactivity and lack of stimulation may provoke atrophy and degeneration of the intact areas of the brain.
- However inappropriate stimulations may stimulate healthy competitor circuits and may hinder functional recovery.
- Impaired cognitive function may have hindering effect on neurogenasis activities and may fail to optimise functional recovery after a stroke.
- It is therefore essential to identify the existence of cognitive defect and adapt rehabilitation to optimise functional recovery.

III

Functional Architecture of the Nervous System that Mediates Motor Activities

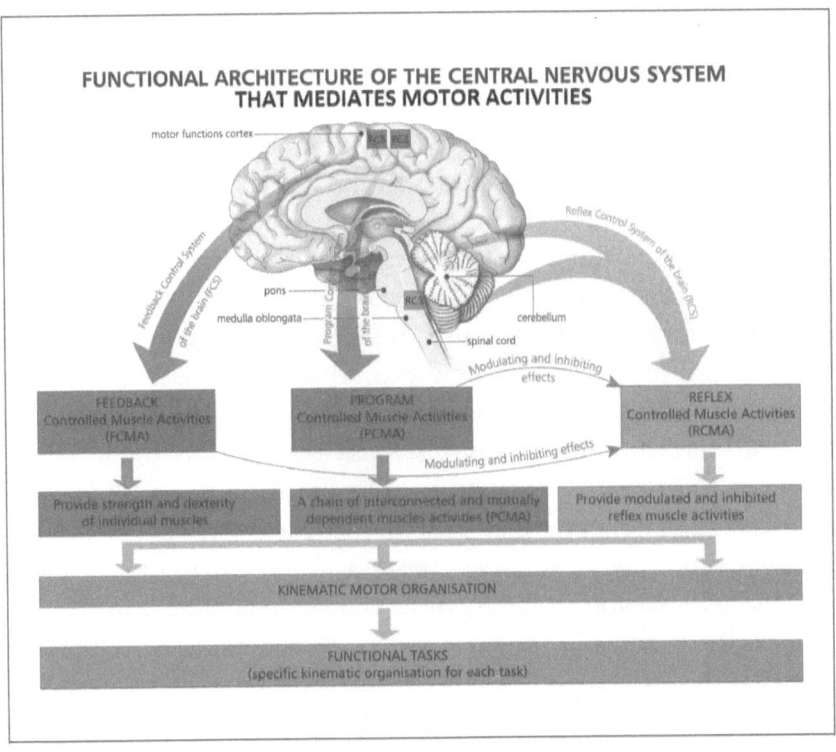

Fig2. A graphic representation of functional architecture of the central nervous system that mediates kinematic motor organisation to perform

different functional tasks. Feedback controlled muscle activities (FCMA) provide individual muscle action; program-controlled muscle activities (PCMA) are chain of multiple muscle activities, they are previously learned and are stored in the brain to be retrieved spontaneously to meet desired functional goal of the performer; reflex-controlled muscle activities provide modulated and inhibited reflex action of muscle.

The ability to move adequately in a continuously changing environment cannot be achieved by individual muscle activity, but it requires an organised kinematic activity of multiple muscles. This kinematic motor organisation consists of a chain of interrelated and mutually dependent muscle activities, which is mediated by neuronal activities within the brain and spinal cord, and which is the result of a combined action of muscle, sensory and cognitive activities. Later on the discussion will elaborate the role of sensory and cognitive function in the mediation of kinematic motor organisation. Moreover the organisational structure constitutes the baseline activity for performing functional task, and each task has its own specific organisational structure, like getting in and out of a chair, getting in and out of a bed or walking, has its specific organisational structure. Moreover the kinematic motor organisation is mediated by a specific motor functional architecture within the central nervous system. This motor functional architecture has a complex role in the process of generation kinematic motor organisation. The neural damage following a CVA is responsible for the damage of this functional organisation. Therefore it is essential to review this architectural structure because only on the basis of adequate understanding of the structure that regulates the motor organisation can one establish the appropriate movement strategies to restore this structure. The objective of the movement strategy is not to improve individual muscle function but to restore the damaged functional structures of the nervous system, so that its role of generating kinematic motor organisation is re-established. In contrast non-specific stimulation may strengthen the non-damaged competitor circuits or it might simply fail to provide the type of precisely shaped stimulation and timed input that is needed to foster changes in a particular lesioned network (Robertson1999).

Several theories have been proposed to explain the functional architecture of the brain that mediates kinematic motor organisation to perform functional activities. One theory proposes that the motor organisation is mediated by three distinct motor controlling systems within the central nervous system. They are program control system, feedback system, and reflex control system. Earlier Mak and Cole (1991) proposed that two major theories need to be considered to explain motor behaviour. A peripheral control model (feedback control) which emphasises the role of sensory feedback in the control of movements has been proposed by Adam (1971) and Adam and Gortz (1973). The other, a central control model (program control), emphasises that a sequence of movements become stored in memory and can be executed without references of feedback (Keel and Posner 1986, Schmidt and Russel 1972). Beside these two motor controlling systems, a third type of motor controlling system, which generates reflex muscle activities which also plays a crucial role in the kinematic organisation of motor activities.

The motor controlling system of the brain that stores previously learned movements, which can be retrieved spontaneously to meet specific functional goal of the performer, is the program control system. Everts and Tanji (1974), and Schmidt (1982) suggest that a rapid task with little requirement of accuracy is mediated by programmed control system. Whereas, the individual muscle activities are mediated by feedback control system of the brain. Moreover the reflex controlled system produces reflex or involuntary muscle activities, which is mainly generated within the brain stem and the spinal cord. During functional task the organised kinematic activities of muscles are the result of combined activity of program, feedback, and reflex controlled muscle activities. In this organisation process the program control system of the brain retrieves a chain of interconnected and mutually dependent muscle activities, the feedback control system provide the strength and dexterity of individual muscles in to these retrieved muscles activities, and finally the reflex control system provides inhibited and modulated reflex muscle activities. In addition these activities are guided and facilitated by different sensory and cognitive functions. It is clear then that the organised kinematic motor activities are not only mediated by muscle activities but also they are the result of a combined action motor, sensory and cognitive function. The following discussion reviews some of the insights of the nervous system's functional architecture that mediate these three motor controlling systems.

II.1 a. Program control system of the brain:

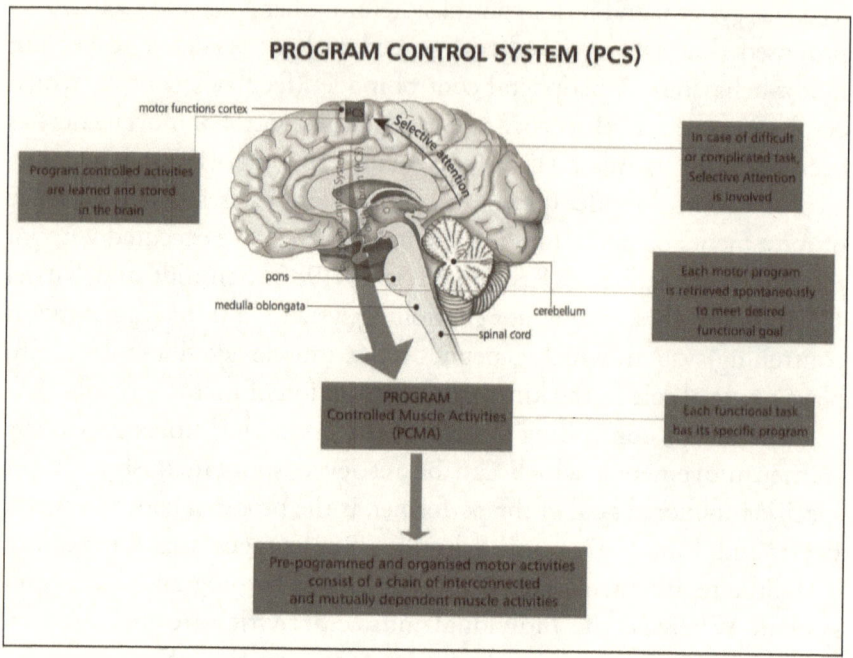

Fig3. Diagram of program control system showing that they consist of a chain of interconnected and interdependent muscle activities. They are previously learned motor activities and are stored as programmed activities, which can be retrieved spontaneously to meet desired goal of the performer. Program-controlled muscle activities (PCMA) play most crucial role in the kinematic organisation of motor activities during functional tasks. Moreover, they exert inhibiting and modulating effect on the reflex controlled muscle activities.

The program control system of the brain uses the sensory, motor, and cognitive function to generate previously learned or programmed muscle activities. Carter and Shapiro (1984), Schmidt (1975) suggest that the centrally controlled movements are governed by generalised motor programs. Keel and Posner (1986), Schmidt and Russel (1972) stated that the program control system of the brain regulates spontaneous and automatic muscle activities. According to Mak and Cole (1991) the generalised motor program view holds that this provides the general characteristics of a movement in response to a variety of environmental demands. They further state that each motor program consists of a set of motor commands specifying the order, timing and amount of muscle contraction necessary to meet the specific demands of the environment or the desired goal of the performer. Learning motor skills, storing them, and then retrieving as an organised muscle activity are the parts of this system. That is, the program controlled system is responsible for the mediation of previously learned motor activities to meet environmental need or desired goal of the performer. Moreover these organised and previously learned motor activities enable one to perform different functional tasks easily and spontaneously.

The basal ganglia neurons along with the other motor areas are responsible for the storing and retrieving of pre-programmed and organised motor activities. To meet environmental demand or desired goal of the performer the BG neurons are activated, which in turn retrieve a series of interconnected and mutually dependent muscle activities. In fact in the retrieval process BG neurons select and activate one group of muscle while inhabit the other in a priority basis and create a specific and organised motor structure. The structure of this motor organisation consists of a succession of muscle activities, which include static, dynamic, concentric and eccentric muscle activities. Moreover the successful organisation of kinematic activity is resulted not alone by the program control system but also by the contribution of feedback control system, which provides strength and dexterity of individual muscle, and the reflex control system which provides the modulated and inhibited reflex activity.

Seitz (1992) and Jueptner et al (1997) both suggest that in the early stages of skill acquisition, frontal cortical regions are used to control movements using attentional processes. With practice, control is relegated to the basal ganglia allowing movements to be executed quickly, easily and automatically (Holden et al 2006, Galletly and Brauer 2005, Jueptner et al 1997). Keele and Posner (1968), and Schmidt and Russell (1972) suggest that in the program control system, the sequence of movement becomes stored in memory and can be executed without reference to feedback. However when a specific response is required, certain parameters are added to the generalised motor program to specify the details of the movement (Mak and Col 1991). These added parameters depend on the feedback control system (a more detailed description of this feedback control muscle activities are discussed in the chapter feedback controlled activities). Getting in and out of a law chair than usual chair or walking on an uneven surface extra muscle effort is required, those extra efforts are provided by feedback control system. However, despite its spontaneous nature, a series of events take place within the brain in the organisation process, while initiating, retrieving and executing of neural activities into programmed muscle activities. According to Marsden (1984) the events include; - goal identification or stimulus to move; -formulation and organisation of motor program; - initiation of movement and finally; - execution of movement. In the above sequence of events the selective attention plays a major role. In other words the internal decision making process in the kinematic organisation of motor activities is mediated by the selective attention. A task of daily living, a routine task for example, less the involvement of attention function is required; however as the task is complicated, walking in an unknown or uneven terrain, the role of selective attention plays crucial role in retrieving and structuring the interrelated and interdependent muscle activities. In fact the selective attention functions as a "clearinghouse" that accumulate samples of ongoing cortical activities and, on a competitive basis, can facilitate any one and suppress others (Luria 1973; Denny-Brown and Yanagisawa 1976). This view is based on clinical evidence presented by Damasio and Colleagues (1980), which demonstrates that lesion in the basal ganglia, may cause unilateral neglect, or hemi-inattention in human. They concluded that the basal ganglia, in combination with frontal and parietal cortical areas, comprise a system sub-serving attention. Therefore selective attention has important role in selection of specific movement program required to achieve desired functional goal. Moreover initial goal identification, then changing goal to adapt according to specific demand of the environment, the executive function plays an important role.

To restore program control system it is essential that whole movement pattern is learned. Since motor skills have a specific organisational structure, they should not be arbitrarily be broken into part for practice, moreover better and more efficient remembering and learning will result from keeping the component of a movement sequence that are interrelated and dependent on each other Hochstenbach and Mulder (1999). Moreover the brain is designed to store the complete program of the movement rather than an individual muscle action. Hochstenbach and Mulder (1999) states that total movement patterns are remembered better than isolated movement. Individual muscle action constitutes irrelevant information for the brain, and may be unattended to be stored in the brain and therefore the relearning of motor function may not be achieved. In contrast a complete program of the movement constitutes the part of relevant information for the brain. The relevant information are attended, and learning is facilitated to be stored in the brain, which are then available to be retrieved in response to the environmental demand or desired goal of the performer.

One evident consequence of a CVA is that the program control system of the brain is impaired, consequently the program controlled activities are either difficult to be executed or they are not available at all for execution. Therefore restoration of impaired program control system constitutes an appropriate strategy to achieve functional goals. In contrast strengthening individual muscles may not be able to restore program control system in the brain. Though, it is obvious that strength and dexterity of individual muscle is essential for the successful organisation of program controlled activities. Similarly inhibiting spasticity may not be able to restore impaired program control system. In contrast the restored program controlled activities can exert modulating and inhibiting effect on spasticity.

In conclusion, the program controlled system is the part functional architecture of the brain that controls functional activities. This system is responsible for the spontaneous and automatic execution of learned muscle activities during functional tasks. The kinematic organisation of motor activities in different functional tasks is largely mediated by the program controlled system. These activities are not the result of pure muscle function but a combined effect of muscle, sensory and cognitive activities is essential for their generation. Moreover human brain is designed for storing the total program of movement rather than storing isolated movement. During early stage of skill acquisition, the program controlled tasks like walking, getting in and out of the bed, getting and out of a chair are learned and stored in the brain by repeated practice and by using conscious voluntary efforts. They are then available for automatic retrieving and executing. In addition these activities exert inhibiting and modulating effect on different reflex muscle activities; therefore an impairment of programmed muscle activities may aggravate different reflex muscle activities. Therefore it is essential to restore the impaired program control system of the brain which in turn can help to mend the broken kinematic organisation of muscle activities following a CVA.

II.1b. Feedback control system of the brain:

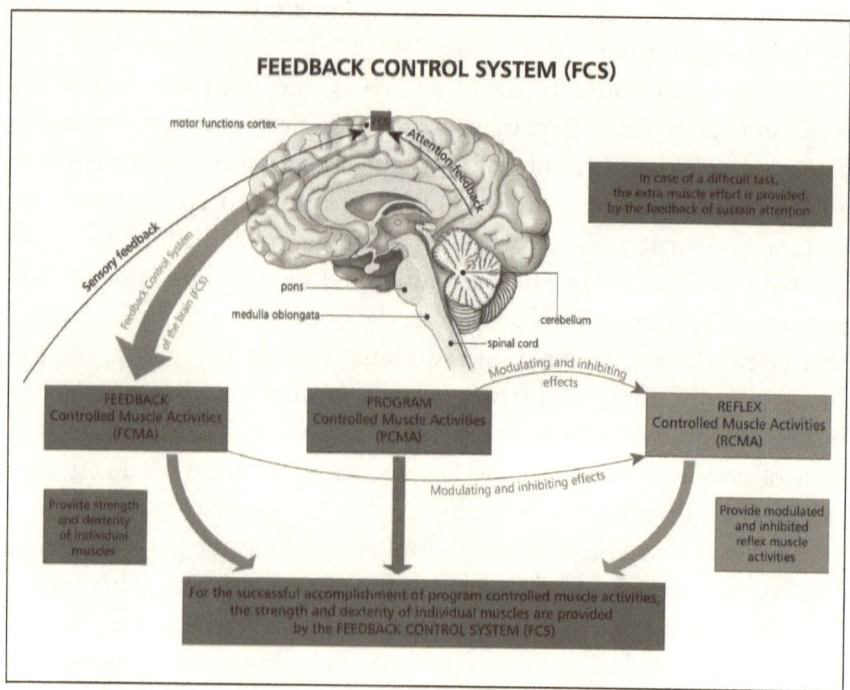

Fig4. Feedback control system provide strength and dexterity of individual muscle while generating kinematic organisation of motor activities. Moreover, they provide inhibiting and modulating effect on th reflex control muscle activities.

Feedback control system generates individual muscle activities, which is the part of motor functional architecture that mediates kinematic motor organisation. Feedback controlled muscle activities are responsible the strength and dexterity of individual muscle that is necessary for the successful execution of program controlled activities. These individual muscle activities are generated in response to sensory feedback received by the motor neurons within the brain. Adams (1971) and Adams and Goetz (1973) stated that in the feedback control model the sensory function plays main role in the control of movements. According to Schmidt (1980) in a feedback controlled activity each mode of control is operational for certain kind of responses or at certain times within a response. For example, a task which has a longer movement duration, or requires a higher degree of accuracy and attention appears to be under feedback control (Keele and Posner 1968, Klapp 1975, Schmidt 197). That is in a routine task, the sensory feedback determines the strength and dexterity of individual muscle; however, when a task requires extra effort, walking on an unknown environment, for example, the feedback from attention function is involved to generate the extra effort. Therefore the feedback controlled activities are the result of a mixed sensory and voluntary effort. The voluntary effort is provided by the attention function. It is then clear that not only sensory feedback but also attention feedback is crucial in the generation of the strength and dexterity of individual muscles. In particular the sustained attention is involved in providing the extra parameter require in the kinematic motor organisation of a difficult task. Unlike selective attention which reflects our capacity to select one stimulation source from among others, the sustained attention reflects the ability to concentrate on a given task over a longer and generally unbroken period of time (More detailed discussion is made on the chapter on Cognitive impairment and relearning of motor function following stroke). Routine functional tasks like getting out of a chair are largely mediated by program controlled activity, and the strength and dexterity of individual muscle is generated as a result of sensory feedback; however in getting out of a low chair when an extra effort is needed; the feedback controlled activities the sustain attention function is involved to add the extra parameter. Program controlled muscle activities are the result of spontaneous muscle action, in contrast feedback muscle activities are resulted from sensory function and conscious and voluntary effort (sustained attention).

Each functional task is the result of an organised kinematic motor activities, this organisational structure consists of a chain of interrelated and mutually dependent muscle activities, which is the function of program control system; moreover each muscle of the interrelated and mutually dependent kinematic motor structure requires a certain strength and dexterity so that the task is successfully executed; which are provided by the feedback control system; and finally the modulated and inhibited reflex muscle activities also contribute to shape the organisation of kinematic motor structure.

Feedback control system may be impaired in a CVA, and people with hemiplegia may be unable to generate the feedback controlled activities. Consequently they will experience difficulty to execute movements using voluntary and conscious effort. Moreover due to lack of strength and dexterity of individual muscle, hemiplegic subject with impaired feedback control system will experience difficulty to perform program control activities. However restoring feedback controlled system or improving strength and dexterity of individual muscle alone may not help improve task performance, unless a simultaneous strategy to restore program control system is also undertaken. In addition, in an impaired feedback control system of the brain, the weakness and loss of dexterity of individual muscle will be unable to exert their inhibiting and modulating effects on different reflex muscle activities.

In conclusion cerebral feedback system provides strength and dexterity of individual muscle in the generalised motor program. They also provide the added parameter or an extra force in performing a difficult task. Normal sensory function is adequate in generating feedback control activities, however when added parameter is needed in performing a difficult task the sustain attention gets involved. Therefore impaired feedback control system will result in a failure to provide the strength and dexterity of individual muscles necessary for the successful execution of program controlled activities; moreover the extra parameter for a difficult task will also be impossible. In addition this system has inhibiting and modulating effect on the spinal and brain stem reflex activities, and its impairment may result in an exaggeration of different reflex activities. Therefore it is important to restore impaired feedback control system, which in turn can help to mend the broken kinematic organisation of motor activities.

III.2. Reflex control system:

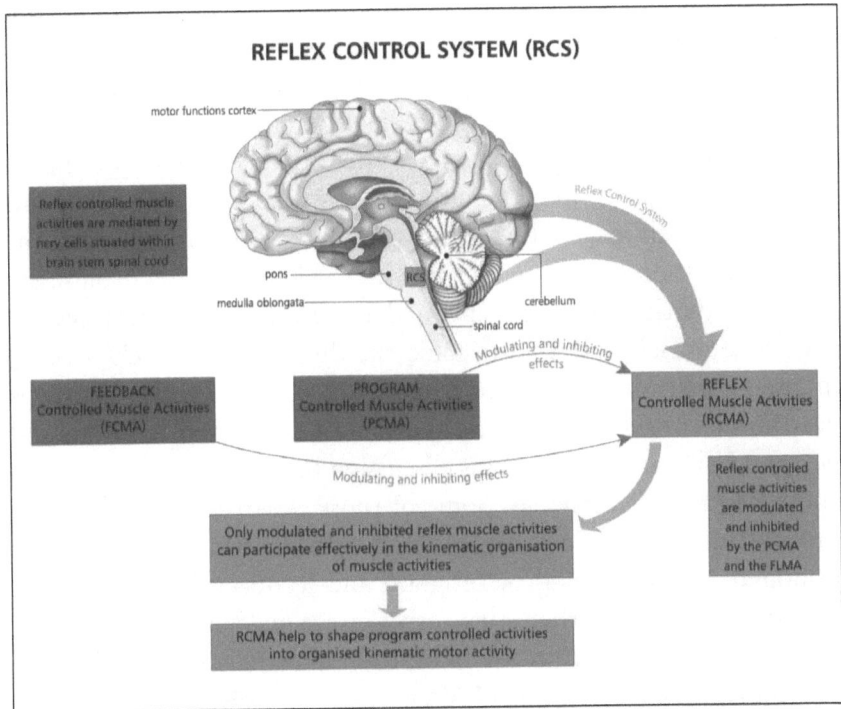

Fig 5. The diagram of reflex control system, which generates reflex muscle activities; they are modulated and inhibited by the program (PCMA) and feedback (FCMA) controlled muscle activities. Only inhibited and modulated muscle activities are effectively participate to produce organised kinematic motor activities.

The third system of motor functional architecture of the brain is the reflex control muscle system. These reflex muscle activities are mostly generated by the spinal cord and the brain stem of the central nervous system. Moreover they function independently, without involvement of higher motor areas. However the reflex muscles activities are only effective to participate in the kinematic organisation of muscle activities when they are modulated and inhibited by program and feedback controlled activities. That is the inhibited and modulated reflex muscle activities constitute the purposeful muscle reflex, whereas uninhibited and non-modulated muscle reflex are the part of involuntary muscle activities and unable to participate in structure of a kinematic motor organisation. For example during walking the extension of knee joint, which is mediated by the quadriceps, when reached to certain extent the stretch reflex of the hamstring muscle produces its contraction to prevent hyperextension of the knee to execute an effective heel strike.

The areas of the central nervous system that control reflex muscle activities are usually remain intact in a stroke. Moreover they are deprived of their modulating and inhibiting effect from the program and feedback controlled motor activities. Therefore the involuntary muscle activities that are generated by the reflex control system and these muscle activities become the dominating muscle activity following a stroke. There are three main types of reflex activities need to be considered, they are spinal reflex, postural reaction, and postural reflex and the following discussion briefly reviews those reflex controlled muscle activities. Some of those reflex activities function to facilitate the kinematic organisation of motor activities, others are inhibited and modulated by program and feedback back controlled activities. Given that the reflex activities are generated as a result of neuronal activities within the brain stem and the spinal cord, those activities are often spared in a CVA.

III 2a. Spinal reflex:

The spinal reflex is the most basic neural circuit, which consists of muscle receptors, their central connections with spinal cord neuron, and the motor-neuronal output to muscle. This neural arc is also considered as lower motor neuron (LMN). The neurons connecting the brain and the spinal cord is considered as upper motor neurons (UMN) and the neurons connecting the spinal cord and the muscle fibres are considered as lower motor neurons (LMN). The lower motor neurons produce spinal reflex. Any stimulation at the level of spinal receptor may provoke spinal reflex activities, which may out of voluntary control of individual. The LMN is the most basic neural circuit, which consists of muscle receptors, their central connections within spinal cord neurons, and the motoneuronal output to the muscles (Katz and Raymer1989). These authors further state that within this arc, the alpha motor neuron may be linked to a final conduit for motoneural outflow, and this outflow is the summation of the host of different synaptic and modulatory influences, including excitatory postsynaptic potentials from group Ia an II muscle spindle afferents, inhibitory post synaptic potential from interneuronal connections from antagonist muscles, and pre-synaptic inhabitation initiated by descending fibre input. For example during walking the contraction of the quadriceps produces the extension of the knee joint and when the extension attain its maximum level the antagonists hamstring stretch receptors produces reflex contraction in order to stop further extension of the knee. Moreover the descending fibres not only exert an inhibiting effect on the reflex arc but also modulate the exaggerated reflex activities into a purposeful functional task. Stroke produces an upper motor neuron (UMN) lesion whereas the lower motor neuron (LMN) remains intact and therefore it can continue to produce involuntary reflex activities.

III.2b. Brain stem reflex:

Another group of reflex activities which are necessary for balance and postural control are generated by the lower part of the brain mainly by the brain stem. Majority of cases after the stroke most of these reflex activities remain intact. These brain stem reflexes are postural reaction and postural reflex activities, and the following discussion review these two reflex activities.

Postural reactions:

Postural reactions are reflex muscle activities necessary to maintain upright posture and they constantly work to readjust upright position of the body. Bobath (1994) affirms that normal postural reflex activity forms the necessary background for normal movement and functional activities. The author further suggests that postural reactions are active movements, although they are subcortically controlled and automatic. The postural reactions include righting reactions, equilibrium reaction, and associated reaction. Bobath (1994) has given the following descriptions regarding righting reactions, equilibrium reaction and associated reaction,

> The righting reactions are automatic reactions which serve to maintain and restore the normal position of the head in the space and its normal relationship with the trunk, together with the normal alignment of trunk and limbs. These reactions develop in the growing infants, are gradually modified and become integrated into more complex activities, such as the equilibrium reactions and voluntary movement, and are essential in the building up of motor patterns for adult life. Throughout the life they are necessary for getting out of the bed, for sitting up, for kneeling down, etc.
>
> Equilibrium reactions are automatic reactions which serve to maintain and restore balance during all our activities, especially when we are in danger of falling. Their development gradually overlaps with those of the righting reactions. Changes at the centre of gravity necessitate continuous postural adjustments during any movement and even the smallest change of tonus has to be countered by changes of tonus throughout the body musculature. If there are considerable displacements of the centre of gravity as, for instance, when there is a danger of falling, the equilibrium reactions are counter-movements of varying ranges to restore threatened balance.

Automatic adaptation of muscles to changes of posture: These automatic reactions can be observed in trunk and limbs, and they overlap to some extent with the equilibrium reactions. A normal postural tone must be high enough to resist gravity, but be low enough to way to movement. Synergic fixation proximally to allow for selective mobility of more distal segments. Automatic adaptation of muscles and postural changes. Graded control of agonists and antagonists integrated with that of synergists for the timing and direction of movement. – The automatic movement patterns of the righting and equilibrium reactions which are the background against which voluntary functional activity takes place.

Postural reflex:

There are several postural reflexes, which help to maintain posture and facilitate the body to adapt in constant change of position during different functional activities. Postural adjustments occur not only as a result of sensory feedback in response to perturbation, but also as a result of 'feed forward' in anticipation of unexpected, self generated perturbation (Horak 1987). Most of the postural reflexes are controlled by lower part of the brain and the brain stem. These postural reflexes are normal reflex, these reflex are the dominating muscle activities in new born, progressively with the development of programmed and feedback controlled muscle activities these reflex activities become no dominating muscle activities. Nevertheless they constantly work to maintain balance and muscle tone. Bobath (1994) describes that in the hemiplegic patient the main factors of abnormal postural reflex activity interfering with movement are:

- Associated reactions
- The asymmetric tonic neck reflex
- The positive support reaction

Associated reactions have been described as tonic reflexes that is tonic postural reaction of muscles deprived of voluntary control (Walshe 1923). In hemiplegic patient, associated reactions produce a widespread increase of spasticity throughout the whole of the affected side (Bobath 1993). Nathan (1980) describes that some of the reactions are the excessive activity of the motor neurones, the increased muscle tone, and the low threshold and prolonged responses to all stimuli. Moreover associated sections may result from any difficulty patient experiences as, for example, fear of falling due to lack of balance, of being agitated when meeting strange people (Bobath 1993). Associated reaction may exaggerate spastic pattern of muscles. Moreover according to (Bobath 1993) the reinforcement and strengthening of the spastic patterns through associated reactions can lead to in time to contracture and deformity.

Asymmetric tonic neck reflex: The asymmetric tonic neck reflex is one of the primitive reflexes, where the movements of the limbs are provoked by the movement of the head. The asymmetric tonic neck reflexes, like associated reactions, are deprived of higher cortical control.

It is present as dominating reflex at birth, however progressively with the development of program and feedback controlled activities their domination minimises. Walshe (1923) found the reaction to be more pronounced if the patient turned his head actively and more so if the rotation is carried out with force against gravity. In many cases, usually those with severe spasticity, the reaction proper cannot be observed and though changes of tone may occur, they are not marked enough to result in a visible movement (Bobath 1993).

Positive support reaction: The positive supporting reaction is the static modification of the spinal extensor thrust, which is a brief extensor reaction, evoked by a stimulus of sudden pressure of the pads of the foot and affecting all the extensor muscles of the limb with relaxation of the antagonists (Sherrington 1947). The positive supporting reaction is characterised by the simultaneous contraction of flexors and extensors (Bobath 1993).

IV. Conclusion: Normal muscle function is the result of neural activities within the brain and spinal cord. Three distinct muscle controlling system is responsible for the generation of an organised kinematic activity of muscles, which enables one to move adequately in a continuously changing environment. They are program control system, feedback control system and reflex control system. In the program controlled model the sequence of movements become stored in memory and can be executed without references of feedback controlled activity (Keel and Posner 1986). The program control system generates interrelated and interconnected muscle activities, which have an organisational structure, and which are specific for each function. In program control system the movements are automatic and spontaneous, usually the whole program is learned and stored in the brain and they are retrieved and executed as a whole program. Feedback control system use sensory feedback to provide the strength and dexterity of individual muscle into the feedback controlled activities. Adam (1971) and Adam and Gortz (1973) had proposed that the peripheral control model (feedback control) emphasises the role of sensory feedback in the control of movements. However when an extra effort is needed, a difficult task per example, the feedback of sustain attention is used to facilitate muscle contraction. The reflex control system provides modulated and inhibited reflex activities.

These three motor controlling systems, which are dependent on each other, constitute the functional architecture of brain and are essential for generating organised kinematic motor activities, and which enable one to move adequately in a continuously changing environment.

Kinematic organisation of motor activities to achieve dynamic adaptation within the environment:

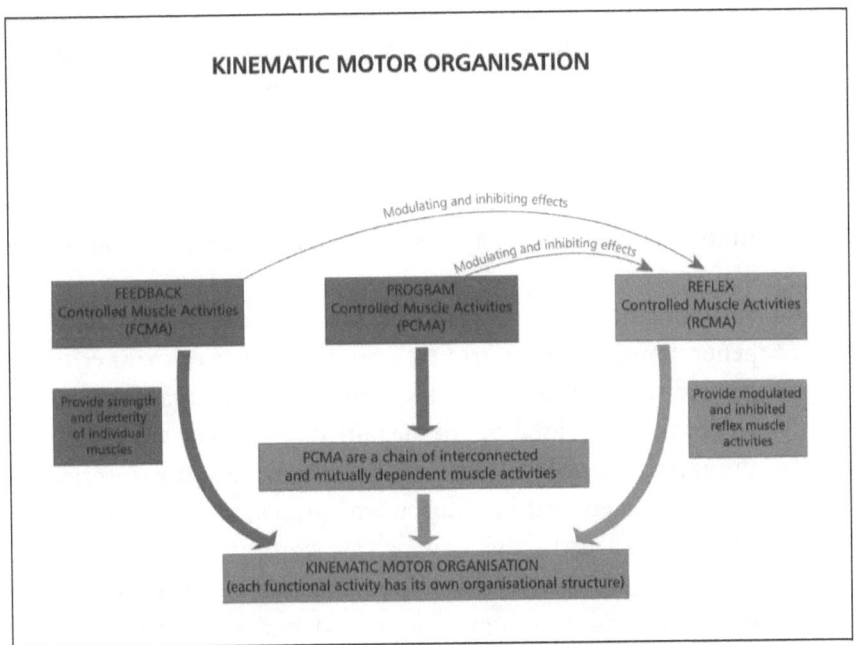

Fig.1. Diagram showing how three distinct motor controlling systems function to mediate kinematic motor organisation. Each functional task has its specific organisational structure

Program control system of the brain launches pre-programmed motor activities, which consist of series of interconnected and interrelated muscle activities. In fact these activities are stored in the basal ganglia. BG functions as a sorting department retrieve the muscle activities and send signal to the cortical motor areas. In this process BG neurons play an important role, which prioritise one action and while suppress other in order to achieve desire functional goal.

However when an extra parameter is requires the feedback control system gets involve and in achieving functional goal.

Summary of the functional architecture of the brain that mediate the kinematic organisation of motor activities:

- Motor neural activities within the brain and spinal cord generate muscle activities that enable one to move adequately in a continuously changing environment.
- Three distinct muscle controlling systems, which generate an organised kinematic activity of muscles, include feedback control system, program control system, and reflex control system.
- The feedback control system of the brain produces individual muscle activities, which provide strength and dexterity of individual muscle in the overall kinematic organisation motor activity.
- In a normal routine task the sensory feedback is used to generate feedback controlled activities, however extra effort is needed in the generation of kinematic motor organisation, the feedback is provided by the sustained attention.
- Program control systems of the brain sets off a series of interconnected and interdependent muscle activities. They are previously learned activities which are stored within the brain as a whole program and retrieved spontaneously as a whole program.
- Reflex control system provides modulated and inhibited reflex activity in the kinematic motor organisation. Reflex activities are involuntary muscle activities, they became purposeful and become part of kinematic organisation of motor activities when they are modulated and inhibited.
- Moreover the inhibition and modulation effects are imposed upon reflex muscle activities by the program and feedback controlled activities.
- The program controlled activities produce automatic and spontaneous muscle activities. These activities are stored in the brain as a whole program, and can be retrieved and executed easily and automatically to achieve a desire goal of the performer or to meet environmental demand.

- Different motor skills like walking, getting in and out of the bed, getting in and out of a chair are largely mediated by programmed controlled activities.
- However when an extra effort is needed, like walking in an uneven surface or unknown environment for example, the parameters are added to the generalised motor program by using feedback control system to specify the details of the movement.
- The reflex system is responsible for a wide range of reflex muscle activities, which are generated mainly by the brain stem and spinal cord.
- Both the program controlled and feedback controlled activities exert inhibiting and modulating effect on the spinal and brain stem reflex activities.
- In stroke, the program controlled and the feedback controlled system of the brain are impaired; consequently hemiplegic subjects experience difficulty or in severe case inability to perform voluntary muscle activities and to perform different functional tasks.
- In contrast, the brain stem reflex and spinal reflex activities remain intact following a stroke, given that the reflex activities are deprived of modulating and inhibiting effects from the feedback and program controlled systems, they become the dominating muscle activities after the stroke.

IV

Consequence of Stroke on the Motor Controlling System of the Brain

The previous discussion has elaborated that three distinct systems of the brain are responsible for the generation of kinematic organisation of motor activities, which enable one to move adequately in a continuously changing environment. Following a CVA, the motor neuronal damage is responsible for the breakdown of the structure of this motor organisation. Before elaborating the strategies to restore this structure, it is useful to review some of the insights of this organisational breakdown. The breakdown of the kinematic motor organisation is mainly due to impairment of two major systems, which are program and feedback control system of the brain. Whereas the reflex control system usually remains undamaged. Moreover in the absence of these two main motor controlling systems the intact reflex control system is deprived of their modulating and inhibiting effects, and uninhibited and non-modulated reflex activities or the spasticity can become the dominating muscle activity following a CVA. However the reduction of reflex muscle activities may not restore program and feedback control system in the brain, unless a precisely shaped stimulation is provided for their restoration is provided. In contrast given that the program control and feedback control systems are impaired, the rehabilitation intervention has to try to restore those two impaired systems. Therefore identifying the motor consequences that result from the impairment of those two systems seem essential to deliver an appropriate intervention. The following discussion reviews the consequences of impaired feedback and program controlled activities, as well as their repercussion on reflex activity of muscle.

Impaired programme control system of the brain:

The program control system is responsible for the generation of previously learned movements, which consist of a chain of interconnected and interdependent muscle activities. Moreover these interconnected and interdependent muscle activities have organisational structure, which is specific for each functional task. In CVA due to an impaired program control system of the brain, the organised activities are no longer available for automatic execution. The basic tasks like getting in and out of the bed, getting in and out of a chair walking within home are largely mediated by the program controlled activities. Not only these basic tasks but also the other learned activities are dependent on the program control system. However it is important to realise that a functional tasks is not the result of a pure motor activity but it is the result of a combined action of cognitive, sensory and motor action. Moreover the strength and dexterity of individual muscle, which are mediated by feedback control system of the brain, as well as modulated reflex activities, are essential for the successful accomplishment of program controlled activities. In addition the program controlled muscle activities exert inhibiting and modulating effect on the reflex muscle activities. Given that different functional tasks are largely mediated by the program controlled muscle activities, relearning of functional tasks therefore seems to be the appropriate intervention to restore the program control system in the brain.

IV.1. Impaired feedback control system of the brain:

The feedback controlled system uses voluntary control mechanism of the brain to produce individual muscle action. Weakness and loss of dexterity of individual muscle is the consequence an impaired feedback controlled system. In extreme cases there may be paralyses muscles, that is, inability to produce muscle contraction event with a voluntary effort. According to Carr and Shepherd (2004) a neural lesion in which motor commands to the muscles are deficient result in decreased strength, even paralysis. The execution of interconnected and interdependent muscles, which are part of program controlled activity, will be difficult, due to the weakness and loss of dexterity of individual muscle. Consequently hemiplegic subjects may experience difficulty to perform functional task or they may tend to perform tasks using compensatory movements. Moreover the weakness and loss of dexterity of individual muscle may unable to exert their inhibiting and modulating effect on the reflex muscle activities. In contrast inhibition or minimising spasticity may not automatically improve strength and dexterity of individual muscles. Appropriate and active exercises of individual muscle, which in turn facilitate restoration of the feedback control system of the brain, can only improve strength and dexterity of individual muscles. The following discussion examines the mechanism of weakness and loss of dexterity of muscles as well as the repercussions of weakness on the loss of dexterity on functional activities.

Muscle weakness:

Feedback control system provides strength of individual muscle, which is essential for the successful execution of program controlled activities. Normally the production of muscle force depends upon the number and type of motor units recruited and the characteristics of both the motor unit discharge and the size of the muscle itself (Carr and Shepherd 2004). Intact descending inputs are necessary for shaping complex movements by graded activation of coordinating muscles and for bringing motor neurons to the high frequency discharge necessary sustained contraction strength (Landau 1988). That is, for muscles to produce the force required to carry out a goal directed action, a necessary number of muscle fibres must contract simultaneously and the various muscle involved in the action must coordinate their force production specific to the task and context (Carr and Shepherd 2004). The authors further suggest that the muscle force is augmented by increasing number of active motor unit discharge and the size of the muscle itself. In stroke following a brain lesion there may be a reduction of the number of motor unit available to activate muscle, which in turn causes muscle weakness. Rosenfalk and Andreassen (1980), Gemperline et al (1995) affirm that the interruption of descending pathways following stroke results in a decrease in the motor units activated, decreased firing rate of motor units and impaired motor unite synchronisation.

Moreover following stroke, muscle weakness may arise from two major sources: primarily from the lesion itself, as a result of a decrease in descending input inputs converging on the final motor neuron population, and hence a reduction in the number of motor unit available for recruitment (Carre and Shepherd 2004). The secondary source of weakness arises as a consequence of lack of muscle activity and immobility (Cruz –Martinanez 1984, Farmer et al 1993). Therefore the strategy to improve muscle function is bilateral; that is, in the one hand it is essential to restore impaired neural function and on the other hand to prevent the development of secondary changes of muscles.

Loss of dexterity: Another muscle dysfunction that appears as a result of an impaired feedback system is the loss of dexterity, and which can be aggravated due to lack of muscle activity. Dexterity is the ability to perform a motor task in a coordinated manner (Carr and Shepherd 2004). The authors further suggest that in loss of dexterity there are decreased number of motor neurons are activated, moreover decreased firing rate and impaired motor unite synchronisation lead to disorganisation of motor outputs at segmental level and underlie motor control problem. Loss of dexterity appears to result from deficits in the sustained and rapid transfer of sensoriomotor information between cerebral cortex and spinal cord (Darien-Smith et al 1996). Lack of consistency in timing and modulating muscle activation may be a cause of the decreased coupling between muscle activation and target movement reported when stroke patients attempted a flexion-extension elbow movement to track a target with low friction manipulation (Canning et al 2000). However at the neurophysiological level, the relationship between muscle strength (generation of appropriate force) and dexterity (coordination of muscle activation) is unclear. Loss of dexterity appears to involve the loss of coordination of muscle activity to meet task and environmental requirements through an impaired ability to fine tune coordination between muscles (Kautz and Brown 1998). Although impaired dexterity is typically considered in its association with weakness and slowness to contract muscle, there is some evidence that they may be independent phenomena (Canning et al 2000). Since rate of transmission from the cortex to spinal cord affects dexterity (Darien-Smith et al 1996), individuals following stroke may have difficulty adapting to the reduce number of corticospinal inputs, having to relay also on slower and less direct corticobulber channels for relaying information (Canning et al 2000). Loss of dexterity of individual muscle can have hindering effect on regaining functional autonomy. Carr and Shepherd (2004) suggest that improved force production and coordination of muscle activity according to task and contextual requirement are both required for effective motor performance.

The brain lesion may result in an impaired feedback controlled system. The feedback controlled system is responsible for the production of individual muscle action. Impaired feedback system is responsible for the weakness and loss of dexterity of individual muscle. Weakness and loss of dexterity of individual muscle can have hindering effect on performing different functional tasks. However strengthening individual muscle and improving its dexterity may not automatically improve the ability to perform different tasks. Moreover due to the weakness and loss of dexterity of individual muscle, the muscles may no longer able to exert inhibiting and modulating effect on brain stem and spinal reflex activities. Consequently there may be uninhibited and exaggerated reflex activity or spasticity. It is therefore important to design rehabilitation strategy to restore the feedback controlled system.

Uninhibited and non-modulated reflex muscle activities:

During functional tasks, in the kinematic motor organisation, the modulated and inhibited reflex muscle activities provide an essential contribution. Program and feedback control systems are damage in a CVA, however the reflex control system of the brain and spinal cord is often remain undamaged. Moreover the intact reflex activities are deprived of the modulating and inhibiting effect from the program controlled and feedback controlled activities. Consequently an uninhibited and non-modulated reflex activity of muscles or spastic movement pattern becomes dominating movement following a CVA. Spastic movement pattern are not the part of the structural entity kinematic motor organisation, and therefore cannot participate effectively in a functional task, in contrast inhabited and modulated muscle reflex constitute the purposeful reflex activities, which in turn effectively contribute to the structuring of organised kinematic activity of muscles. However the efforts to reduce spasticity may have very little effect in improving functional activity level; given that a reduced spasticity cannot participate in the structure of kinematic motor organisation. In contrast the restored program and feedback control systems effectively can exert their modulating and inhibiting effect on the uncontrolled muscle reflex and transform them into purposeful muscle reflex, which in turn can effectively participate in the structure of kinematic motor organisation.

Consequences of CVA on motor controlling system include an impaired program control and feedback control system of the brain, with an undamaged reflex control system. Program and feedback control system largely contribute to the generation of kinematic organisation motor activities in performing functional tasks. Whereas the feedback control system provides the strength and dexterity of individual muscle that is necessary to execute program controlled activities. Moreover these two systems exert modulating and inhibiting effect on the reflex controlled activities.

Kinematic organisation of muscle activities in different functional tasks:

The understanding of the kinematic organisation of program controlled activities is therefore essential to undertake appropriate strategy to be undertaken to relearning those tasks.

Sit to stand difficulty in people with hemiplegia:

Standing up from a chair is a task that is performed many times every day by normal adults, including the aged (Ada and Westwood (1992). Aniansson et al (1980) report that 94 per cent of healthy 70-year-olds have no difficulty standing up from an normal dining chair without using their arms. Large part muscle activity in standing from sitting is a spontaneous action and generated by program controlled system of the brain. Elderly patients following stroke often have difficulty performing this task, which in turn seriously impairs overall mobility (Ada and Westwood (1992).

Kinematic analysis of sit to stand (STS):

Kinematic analysis of STS demonstrates that it requires translation of body mass in horizontal and vertical direction from a relatively stable sitting position with thighs and feet as base of support, to a period of relative instability when the thighs leave the seat and the feet becomes base of support (Carr and Shepherd 2004). This means while hip and trunk flexors work to bring the trunk forward, the extension of the knees start to lift the thigh off the chair. It is evident from several studies that a timing relationship between the flexion of the trunk at the hip and onset of lower limb extension is a crucial feature in the movement organisation (Pai and Roger 1990, Schenkman et al 1990, Shepherd and Gentile 1994). Although apparently a simple task yet it is the product of complex and synchronised effort of several individual muscles. Clinical observation of attempts to stand up patients following stroke revealed relatively slow movement as well as lack of coordination between hip and knee (Ada and Westwood 1992). These authors further affirm that these patients often complete knee extension while their hips were still extending. Motor impairment along with the presence of sensory impairment, spasticity, weakness of individual muscle, cognitive impairment may further complicate the task difficulty. An important consideration while planning rehabilitation strategy is to re-educate the whole program instead of insisting on improving individual movements. Given that the brain is designed in such a way that it can only store the whole program of movement. However it is equally important to improve individual muscle function, as each task is the combination of multiple individual muscle function.

Summary of kinematic
- Forward flexion of trunk, flexion of hips and flexion of knees
- Stop flexion of the trunk, and start extension (stretch reflex guide to limit trunk flexion)
- Start extension of hips and knees to lift thigh of the chair

Kinematic analysis of walking:

Muscle activities during walking consist of static muscle work as well as dynamic muscle work. Muscles work statically to assure stability of joint, while other muscles work dynamically to provide propulsion of the limb to move forward. This static as well as dynamic muscle activities in turn produce bilateral alternative movements of both lower and upper limbs, dissociation of pelvic and pectoral girdles, and an erected spinal column. Moreover those activities not only hold body in upright position and at the same time shift the body forward but also enable one to adapt and adjust in constant changing position of body as well as constant change of environment. According to Carr and Shepherd (2004) many structural and physiological elements or components cooperate to produce coordinated walking in a changing environment. In addition coordinated walking is obtained 'by linking muscles and joints so that they act together as a single unite or synergy, thus simplifying the coordination of movement' (Bernstein 1967). Sensory system like superficial sensation and deep sensation from different joints of lower limb contributes to smooth and safe walking. Carr and Shepherd (2004) suggest that sensory input in general and visual input in particular provide information that makes it possible for us to walk in varied, cluttered environment and uneven terrains. Given that sensory function has their diverse aspect (e.g. superficial and deep sensation, visual and proprioception) therefore, in case of impairment of one aspect of sensory function, the other aspect of sensory function can help compensate that loss, which in turn enables one to walk despite loss of one of the sensory function. For example impaired visual sensation in case of blindness one can continue to walk, in which case the acuity other sensory functions increase in order to compensate loss of visual sensation. Similarly loss of propioception can be compensated by visual sensation. Therefore it is clear that walking performance requires adequate muscle force, an intact sensory, balance and cognitive function, and impairment of any of these functions may severely jeopardy individual's ability to walk.

An erected static position of the body at the same time propulsion of the body forward is achieved by bilateral and alternative movements of the right and left part of the body. These bilateral alternative movements of lower limbs produce a stance phase and a swing phase; in stance phase the body is supported by one leg, while the other leg swings to move the body forward. According Carr and Shepherd (2004) the gait cycle includes a stance phase (approximately 60%) and a swing phase (approximately 40%). The stance phase can be further subdivided into weight acceptance, mid-stance and push-off, while swing is divided into lift-off (early swing) and reach (late swing) (Winter et al 1987). In-between stance and swing phase, there are two brief period of double support phases. The duration of double support time may increase with aging; that is, as the time spent in double support increases the walking becomes slower, and with the increased of the velocity of walking time spent in double support reduces. Therefore it is clear that intact muscle and sensory functions are essential for walking. Moreover balance reaction is also an important factor for facilitate smooth performance of gait cycle. It is the ability to balance the body mass relative to the base of support that enables us to perform everyday actions, (including walking) effectively and efficiently (Carr and Shepherd 2004). They further state that apart from double support period, the body is in a potentially unstable state. Safe foot clearance and foot contacts are, therefore essential to rebalancing the body mass during double support (Winter et al 1987). With aging process as balance reaction can be weakened, and the elderly subjects may compensate this weakness by increasing double support phase, as well as widening the base of support or the distance between two feet.

Kinematic organisation of motor activities in walking:

Kinematic variables provide information about angular displacements, paths of the body parts and the centre of body mass (CBM), with angular and linier velocities and accelerations (Carr and Shepherd 2006). Normally individual variations in the magnitude of angular displacement are relatively small, with the greatest variances occurring in the less obvious movements of ankle and foot (Sutherland et al 1994). Carr and Shepherd (2006) describe that the mass of the upper body, including pelvis and trunk, responds to the needs of the individual to advance the lower limb and to transfer body weight from one supporting limb to other. For example, the pelvis (moving at the hip joints and joints of the lumbar spine) rotates, tilts, and shifts laterally, governed by such factors as muscle length and length of stride. Shoulders rotate and arm swing out of phase with displacement of pelvis and leg. Moreover while one group of muscles work dynamically the others work statically to assure upright position of the body. During stance phase the body weight is supported by one leg and this supporting is maintained by static work of muscles of trunk, pelvis and lower limb, at the same time muscles of the other side of the body work dynamically to propel the limb forward. According to Carr and Shepherd (2006) the linking muscles and joints act together as a single unit or synergy, thus simplifying the coordination of movement. Walking is complex, whole body action that requires the cooperation of and coordination of a large number of muscles and joints to function together and where many structural and physical elements or components cooperate to meet a changing physical and social environment (Carr and Shepherd 2006).

Bobath (1994) suggests that the aim of treatment should be to inhibit the patient's abnormal pattern of movements because we cannot superimpose normal on abnormal patterns; they should not be reinforced and perpetuated by the effort involved in strengthening the muscles. However according to Carr and Shepherd (2004) clinical research has shown that the effort applied in strengthening training does not increase spasticity (reflex hyperactivity). The statement is based on the clinical research carried out by Butefisch et al (1995), Sharp and Bower (1997), Brown and Kautz (1998) Teixera-Salmela et al (1999), Ada and O'Dwyer (2001), Bateman et al (2001).

Moreover studies by Butefisch et al (1995) Miller and Light (1997), Teixera-Salmela et al (1999), which have suggested that not only does strengthen training result in increased muscle strength following stroke, but also improved functional performance and decreased spasticity, for example decreases in resistance to passive movement, stretch reflex hyperactivity and co-contraction. Nevertheless non-specific stimulation can inadvertently strengthen non-damaged competitor circuits of the brain or it might simply fail to provide the type of precisely shaped and timed input that is needed to foster changes in a particular lesioned network (Robertson 1999). That is, an inappropriate stimulation may further imbalance the delicate balance between reflex activities and inhibiting and modulating effects of program and feedback controlled activities. Therefore the objective of the strengthening the muscles is to facilitate recovery of the impaired feedback and program controlled system, which can eventually reinstate the balance between different types of muscle activities. In contrast the inhibition of the spasticity may not be able to restore program and feedback controlled system in the brain. It is obvious that during individual muscle exercise the segment and the limb should be placed in an inhibition position in order to minimise the interfering effect of the spasticity during different exercises. The following discussion examines the effects of released spinal reflex, postural reaction and postural reflex.

Uninhibited and non-modulated reflex muscle activities - spasticity:

Muscle function in post stroke hemiplegic is dominated by the presence of abnormal or exaggerated reflex activities of muscle. According to Bobath (1994) the brain lesion 'cuts off' higher integrated activity and releases uncontrolled postural reflex as well as spinal reflex, producing muscle spasticity. The author further suggests that the spasticity and released postural reflexes are underlying factor for the impaired movement; therefore physical intervention should be designed so that people after stroke can learn to inhibit exaggerated reflex activities and facilitate normal movements. The following discussion examines some of the aspects of released spinal as well as other reflex activities, which contributes to muscle spasticity.

Release of spinal reflex:

Spinal reflex is the a part of normal reflex activity of muscles; however the spinal reflex activities are modulated and inhibited by the by program and feedback controlled activities. Moreover only modulated and inhibited refex activities can effectively participate the generation of kinematic organisation of motor activities. The activity of many descending pathways is likely to be impaired in supraspinal injuries, loss of the inhibiting effects of the descending pathways (especially reticulospinal) on regional interneurons receiving input from cutaenous and muscle segmental afferents is also believed to be very important, especially in spinal form of spasticity (Katz and Raymer 1989). The following discussion examines some of the mechanism that is responsible for the spasticity in people with stroke.

Muscle spasticity:

Spastic hypertonia has been defined as a motor disorder characterised by a velocity-dependent increase in tonic stretch reflexes (muscle tone) with exaggerated tendon jerks, resulting from hyperexcitability of the stretch reflex, as one component of upper motor syndrome (Katz et al 1989). A widely accepted definition of spasticity is that of a motor disorder characterised by velocity-dependent increase in tonic stretch reflexes with exaggerated tendon jerks, resulting from the hyperexcitability of the stretch reflexes (Lance 1980). However other uninhibited brain stem reflexes may be added to the spinal reflex, increasing the intensity and complexity of the spasticity. According to Bobath (1991) the spasticity is caused by the release of an abnormal postural reflex mechanism which results in exaggerated static function at the expense of dynamic postural control. That is, the spasticity shows itself in typical patterns produced by interaction of various release tonic reflexes, whereas flaccidity is the result of lack of postural reflex (Bobath 1991). Katz and Rymer (1989) ha sdescribed that the most basic neural circuit contributing to spastic hypertonia is the segmental reflex arc, which consists of muscle receptors, their central connections with spinal neurons, and motor neuron output to muscle. Within this arc, the alpha motor neuron may be linked to a final conduit of motor neuronal outflow. This out flow is the summation of a host of different synaptic and modulatory influences situated within muscle receptors in the spinal neuron and within motor neuron output (Katz and Rymer 1989). They further suggest that it is upon these basic pathways that spinal and supraspinal influences modulate reflex behaviour. The loss of inhibition may arise as a result of direct pathway interruption (as spinal and brainstem injury), of loss of supraspinal facilitation of brainstem, reticulospinal neurons, thus releasing a number of powerful segmental reflexes which are normally completely suppressed (Burk et al 1972, Lance 1980). The lesion, in effect, 'cut off' higher integrated activity and produce abnormal motor output, a kind of 'short circuit' into the released abnormal patterns of spasticity(Bobath 1994). It is then clear, that uncontrolled postural reflex activities added to the uncontrolled spinal reflex only aggravate the spastic pattern of the muscles in people with stroke. Bobath (1994) further suggests that the release of spinal reflex, automatic reaction and abnormal postural reflexes cause abnormal and involuntary movements. Instead of a normal postural tone, we find spasticity; instead of the normal coordination of righting, equilibrium, we find exaggerated postural reflexes.

One important aspect is that the spasticity is non-progressive in post stroke hemiplegia. However increased spasticity is often observed in late stage of hemiplegia. This is mainly due weakness of existing intact muscles as well as shortening of muscle and other tissues. In case of muscle shortening along with shortening of other tissues the threshold for the spasticity will increase, i.e. spasticity of muscle will appear in minimum stimulation. Chapman and Weisendanger (1982) suggest that plastic changes in synaptic connections may contribute to this slow development of increased spasticity. Furthermore Carr et al (1995) describe that an increased and abnormal sensitivity of pre- or post-synaptic elements to remaining afferent input, i.e. increased chemical sensitivity, can possibly contribute to the increased spasticity. Experiment carried out by Dietz et al (1981); Berger et al (1984); Hufschmidt and Mauritz (1985); Carey and Burghardt (1993) have found that changes in the intrinsic muscle mechanical properties (rather than stretch reflex enhancement) are largely responsible for the aggravating spastic hypertonia in the later stage of hemiplegia. Their claims are based on electromyographic and tension analysis of leg muscles during ambulation of hemipligic adults and children with cerebral palsy. Abnormally high tension developed in the spastic triceps surae during passive stretch without a parallel increased in electromyographic activity. Therefore, resistance to passive movement is due not to neural mechanisms but due to changes in mechanical fibre properties of muscle. Carr et al (1995) also affirm this hypothesis and they conclude that the soft tissue adaptations provide a mechanical cause for the increase in resistance to passive movement. Moreover, Katz, et la (1989) describes that the intramuscular and surface EMG recording from spastic patients demonstrate disturbances of spatial selection of hemiparatic limbs. Furthermore, the severity of spasticity can be dependent on the strength of antagonist muscles. For example, spastic lower limb can be in triple flexion even with a little stimulation when the antagonist extensor muscles are weak, whereas if the extensor muscles are strong enough they can counter act the spasticity and thus can prevent the triple flexion of lower limb. Besides weakness, the antagonist muscles can be spastic as well. This simultaneous spasticity of agonist and antagonist muscles can result in a rigidity of the whole limb.

In conclusion spasticity is the exaggerated spinal reflex activities, which is mainly due to lack of inhibiting and modulating effects of the UMN activities. Moreover the spinal reflex activities or spasticity can be further aggravated by the presence of uninhibited postural and automatic reactions (brainstem reflex activities). Spasticity is non-progressive because electromylographic examinations have demonstrated that the intrinsic muscle mechanical properties rather than stretch reflex enhancement are largely responsible for the spastic hypertonia. However increased spasticity observed in the later stage in stroke patients, can be mainly due to the plastic change in the synaptic connections, increased sensitivity of remaining afferent elements, adaptive shortening soft tissues. Moreover, muscle weakness, which may further minimise the inhibiting effects on the LMN which may be responsible for the aggravation of LMN activities.

Conclusion on the consequence of CVA on the motor controlling system of the brain:

The motor neuronal lesion within the brain in a CVA is responsible for impaired muscle function. The underlying factors that are responsible for the motor dysfunction include an impaired program and feedback control system of the brain. Therefore people with hemiplegic will either experience difficulty or unable to produce the program and feedback controlled activities. The program control system is responsible for the spontaneous retrieval of previously learned muscle activities. They consist of a chain of interconnected and interdependent muscle activities. These activities have specific structural pattern, which is again specific for specific task. The strength and dexterity of individual muscle that are necessary for the execution of program controlled activates are provided by the feedback control system of the brain. Feedback control system uses the feedback of sensory stimulation and sustained attention to generate the feedback controlled muscle activities. In a routine task sensory feedback can provide the strength and dexterity of the muscle necessary for the task, however in case of a difficult task the feedback of sustained attention is used to provide the added parameters needed for the task. Moreover reflex control system provides modulated and inhibited reflex activity, which is essential for the kinematic organisation of motor activities. In addition the modulation and inhibition effect on the reflex activities can only be achieved by the activities of the program and feedback control system. These three systems constitute the essential entity for the generation kinematic organisation of motor activities. In CVA, the lesion of motor neurons of the brain impairs the program and feedback control system, often leaving the reflex control system unaffected. Therefore the uninhibited and non-modulated reflex activities or spasticity is often dominating feature in people following a CVA.

Summary of muscle impairment after stroke:

- Brain lesion after stroke is responsible for the impairment of the program controlled and feedback controlled activities; the reflex controlled activities remain intact in stroke but they

are deprived of the modulating and inhibiting effect of the program controlled and feedback controlled activities.
- Impairment of program controlled system: This system is responsible for the automatic and spontaneous muscle activities. In the early stages of skill acquisition, frontal cortical regions are used to control movements using attentional processes (Seitz 1992, Jueptner et al 1997); with practice, control is relegated to the basal ganglia, allowing movements to be executed quickly, easily and automatically (Holden et al 2006, Jueptner et al1997, Galletly and Brauer 2005). Therefore the program controlled system enables one to perform different functional tasks like getting in and out a bed, getting in and out of a chair, walking, easily and automatically. The brain damage after stroke is responsible for the impairment of program controlled or automatic movements leading to difficulty to perform functional tasks and the severity of the functional difficulty depends on the severity of severity of damage of program controlled system.
- Impairment of feedback system: The feedback system plays an important role in the production of conscious voluntary muscle activities. The impairment of voluntary movements results in a weakness and loss of dexterity of individual muscles.
- Weakness and loss of dexterity of individual muscle will render it difficult to perform different functional tasks; however improving individual muscle function may not automatically improve task performances.
- Hemiplegic subjects experience difficulty to perform individual muscle activities; they also are unable to perform different functional tasks.
- It is therefore important to undertake appropriate treatment strategy to restore program controlled system and feedback controlled system of the brain.
- Moreover program control system and feedback control system have inhibiting and modulating effect on the brain stem and spinal reflex activities.
- Uninhibited and non-modulated reflex muscle activities (muscle spasticity): Postural and spinal reflexes are the part

of normal reflex activities; however they are modulated and inhibited by automatic and voluntary movements in order to generate purposeful functional tasks. Therefore in the absence of modulating and inhibiting effects of the automatic and voluntary activities of the muscles, the postural and spinal reflex activities or spasticity may play a dominating role following a stroke.

- Spasticity is not progressive; however adaptive change of muscle and different soft tissues may increase the threshold for the spasticity.

V

Strategy to Restore Impaired Structure of Functional Architecture Central Nervous System that Mediates Kinematic Motor Organisation

As mentioned earlier that three distinct system or structure of motor functional architecture is responsible for the kinematic organisation of muscle activities. And these organised kinematic motor activities are responsible effectively performing different functional tasks. In CVA there is breakdown of this architectural structure occurs, which leads to difficulty to perform different functional tasks. Two main motor controlling systems within the brain's motor functional architecture are impaired; they are program control and feedback control system. Therefore the activities that can restore these two functional structures of the brain can constitute the appropriate stimulation. The appropriate activities to restore impaired motor neural function will not only facilitate the restoration of program and feedback control system in the brain, but also those restored activities will help to shape uncontrolled reflex activities into modulated, inhibited and purposeful reflex activities. These restored activities along with the purposeful reflex activities can help the generation of organised kinematic activities of the muscles. In addition brain damage can be responsible for the associated dysfunctions like impaired sensory, balance and cognitive functions, and these associated dysfunctions can also have interfering effect on the task performance. Therefore rehabilitation strategy will include the restoration of both the programme and feedback controlled systems in the brain, which has to be adapted taking in to account of the associated dysfunctions.

III a. Activities to restore feedback controlled system in the brain:

Feedback controlled system produces individual muscle activities using conscious voluntary effort. Impaired feedback controlled system results in weakness and loss of dexterity of individual muscle or muscle group and in extreme case hemiplegic subjects unable to produce contraction of individual muscle. Strength and dexterity of individual muscle is essential to for the execution of structured and organized kinematic motor activities. Carr and Shepherd (2004) describe this individual muscle activity as the sub-task of the whole organizational structure of motor activity. An important question is determining which component part of the action to practice separately (Carr and Shepherd 2004). For example, if a patient cannot activate planterflexor muscles with the necessary force and at the appropriate time to push-off, repetitive, resisted exercises are necessary to strengthen these muscles; and the practice of sub-task is then incorporated into walking during training (Carr and Shepherd 2004). The individual muscle weakness can help to identify the part of feedback controlling area of the brain is impaired and which is needed restoration. Therefore the activities to restore feedback control system include:

- 1. Individual muscle exercise
- 2. Exercise of muscle chain
- 3. Functional exercise

Individual muscle exercise:

Individual muscle re-education starts as soon as subject's general condition permits. Weakness and loss of dexterity of individual muscle is unable to exert inhibiting and modulating effect on the reflex controlled activities. According to Bobath (1992) individual muscle strengthening is done in a reflex inhibition position. That is, strengthening exercises are done without reinforcing the spastic pattern. It appears, therefore, that reduction of spasticity in treatment makes isolated movement possible, or, that isolated movement reduces spasticity (Bobath1992). Moreover activities in reflex inhibition position hinder the stimulation of healthy competitor neural circuit in the brain. However inhibiting spasticity may not improve the strength and dexterity of individual muscles. In contrast improve strength of muscle can have inhibiting effect on different uncontrolled reflex activities, which in turn will help to reduce spasticity. According to Smith et al (1999) strength training following stroke not only results in increased muscle strength but also improve functional performance and decreased spasticity of muscles. The dynamic stretching that occurs during active exercise may play a part in decreasing muscle hyperexcitability and increasing muscle compliance (Otis et al 1985; Hummelsheim et al 1994).

Different exercises to improve muscle force will enhance muscle excitation capacity, improve rate of recruitment of motor neuron pool, capacity to inhabit agonist muscles, motor unit activation and synchronization and motor firing pattern will also be ameliorated (Hakkinen and Komi 1983, Sale 1987). Moreover strengthening training can enhance stimulation of metabolic, mechanical and structural muscle fiber changes that result in larger and stronger muscles due to an increase in actin and myocin protein filaments (Sale 1987; Thepaut-Mathieu et al 1988). These above effects were found following research on able-bodied individuals, and it seems similar effects may be facilitated in post stroke hemiplegic subjects. A relationship has been reported between increased muscle strength in lower limbs and improved standing balance (Bohannon 1988) and walking speed (Sharp and Bower 1997, Teixeira-Salmela et al1999, 2001). Moreover major impairments limiting motor performance is muscle weakness or paralysis, soft tissue contracture, lack of endurance and physical fitness (Carr and Shepherd 2004). The authors further suggest that major goal of physiotherapy in neurological rehabilitation is the optimisation of functional motor performance. Moreover decreased force of individual muscle is responsible for the difficulty to perform different functional tasks, whereas increased strength of individual muscle may not help to improve function. Rutherford

(1988) suggests that an increasing strength may not be sufficient to bring about improved walking performance without practice of the action itself, which is necessary for neural adaptation to task and context to be regained. Although strengthening may help to improve force, excitability as well as metabolism of muscles but individual muscle strengthening may not be sufficient to alter functional status in people with stroke. However each functional activity is the combination several individual muscle actions, therefore it is natural that the individual muscle function form the basis for the global functional activity. It is therefore reasonable to improve function or strength of individual muscle to facilitate the performance of functional tasks. There seems little doubt that active exercise and training provoke efficacious changes in motor control (Carr and Shepherd 2004). The authors summarised the effects of strengthening training as follows:

1. Muscle weakness is a major impairment to effective functional performance
    - a stroke usually result in some degree of muscle weakness, including paralysis primarily as a direct result of reduction of in descending inputs on the spinal motor neurons and on the number of motor units activated
    - the immobility which ensues results in mechanical and functional changes to the muscles and connective tissues, and predisposes to further reductions in strengthen
    - elderly individuals may have had varying degree of muscle weakness and reduced endurance.

The objective of improving individual muscle function is restore impaired feedback controlled system in the brain.

In addition, different exercises aim to improve individual muscle function helps to provide neural stimulation which intern facilitates neural recovery and restore feedback control system in the brain. In contrast stimulation deprivation may hinder the process of restoration of feedback control system. The next chapter examines the possibility to facilitate neural recovery by improving individual muscle function.

Improve individual muscle function to restore feedback controlled system:

The neuromuscular adaptation associated with muscle strengthening in the able-bodied is due to neural adaptations to neural drive, which are both quantitative (increase neural drive to the target muscles) and qualitative (reduced co-contraction and improve coordination among synergists) (Hakkinen and Komi 1983; Rutherford and Jones 1986; carolan Caarelli 1992; Yue and Cole 1992). Moreover Hakkinen and Komi (1983), Sale (1987) suggest that strengthening training facilitates neuromuscular changes due to reorganised drive from the supraspinal centres; and these changes include:

- Enhanced muscle excitation,
- Improvement in recruitment of motorneuron pool,
- Inhibition of antagonist muscles,
- Motor unit activation and
- Synchronisation of the firing pattern of motor units.

An important objective of motor relearning is to facilitate neural recovery. Appropriate individual muscle help to facilitate changes like;

- Experience-dependent
- Functional reorganisation
- Facilitate maturation newly proliferated neurons
- Inhibit the competitor neural circuits.

According to Carr and Shepherd (2004) although there is mounting evidence indicating that patterns of use affect reorganisation, and increase acceptance of a link between brain reorganisation and recovery of function, it is still not generally accepted in medical or therapy practice that there might be link between specific rehabilitation method and functional recovery. One aspect is clear that motor impairment in stroke is resulted from neural damage; therefore facilitation of neural recovery will only assure motor recovery.

Experience-dependent change: Repeated use of individual muscles in an inhibition position may help to facilitate experience-dependent changes in the intact neural circuits. In contrast non utilisation of individual muscles may be responsible for the experience deprivation and hinder the facilitation of experience-dependent change. Lee and van Donkelaar (1995) describe that the recovery of function occurring early following stroke reflects reparative processes in the peri-infarct zone adjacent to the injury. These include the resolution of local factors such as oedema, absorption of necrotic tissue debris and the opening of collateral channels for circulation to the lesion area. However the presence of an impaired cognitive function may have hindering effect in fostering experience-dependent change in the brain (more discussion is made on the chapter on cognitive function in stroke).

Inhibition of intact competitor circuit: Stimulation of intact competitor circuit has to be avoided while designing rehabilitation strategy. Robertson and Murre (1999) suggest that the way in which neural recovery from brain damage can take place is through the lifting of inhibition over damaged networks by healthy competitor circuits. This can take place either by damping down the inhibition competition or by boosting the activation in circuits in the lesioned network (Robertson 1999). Each exercise is performed in an inhibition position so that the intact neural circuits responsible for the spinal and postural reflex activities are not strengthen. The aim of treatment should be to inhibit the patient's abnormal pattern of movement because we cannot superimpose normal on abnormal patterns (Bobath1994)

Functional reorganisation: Extensive training of individual muscle also helps to facilitate functional reorganisation. For example in case of damaged neural centre of quadriceps muscle; an extensive training to improve quadriceps muscle may facilitate functional reorganisation that is function of quadriceps muscle will be taken over by other intact neural circuits; in contrast stimulation deprivation may be responsible for the propagation of damaged area. However what are the precisely shaped and timely stimulation that can facilitate functional reorganisation is not clear. According to Carr and Shepherd (2004) training and practice using methods that that facilitate motor learning or relearning would be essential to the formation of functional connections in the intact neural circuits. Human studies provide evidence for functional plasticity after stroke associated with meaningful use of a limb involving task oriented repetitive exercise

(Nelles et al 2001). Increase of synaptic efficacy in existing neural circuits in the form of long-term potentiation and formation of new synapses may be involved in earlier stage of motor learning (Asanuma and Keller 1991). While some pioneering researches on rehabilitation have argued that rehabilitation might under certain circumstances have direct neural effects (Bach-y-Rita 1989), the prevailing view has been that rehabilitation following brain damage had its effects by fostering what Luria termed 'functional-reorganisation' of surviving undamaged brain circuits in order to achieve impaired behavioural goals in a different way.

Conclusion:

- Impaired feedback control system in stroke is responsible for the weakness and loss of dexterity of individual muscles.
- People following a stroke with an impaired feedback control system experience either difficulty or inability to produce voluntary muscle activities.
- It is therefore important to improve the function of individual muscles and minimise their weakness and loss of dexterity.
- Individual muscle exercise are done in spastic inhibition position
- Weakness of individual muscle may be responsible for the difficulty to perform different tasks; but improve individual muscle may not improve task performance.
- Re-education of functional tasks without improving individual muscles may be responsible for using compensatory movements.
- Strengthening individual muscle may facilitate neural change like experience-dependent change, functional reorganisation

Example of individual muscle exercise in spastic inhibition position:

Individual muscle exercise can be done in maximum inhibition position then the exercises will be done progressively in less and less inhibition posture. For example spastic pattern of the upper limb is abduction of the scapula, flexion, adduction and internal rotation of the shoulder; flexion of the elbow and pronation of the forearm; flexion of the wrist and the fingers. Therefore the maximum inhibition position will be extension, abduction and rotation extern of shoulder, extension of the elbow, supination of forearm, extension of the wrist and fingers. To start with the exercise of the scapula, shoulder girdle, elbow, and wrist will be done in the maximum inhibition position. Progressively subject has to learn same movement in less inhibition position until she/he is capable of performing movement in normal anatomical position. Moreover each exercise is done in most simple position and progress to more complex position. That is, the exercises are done in lying then in sitting and finally in standing position.

- Mobilisation of the shoulder girdle can be done best in supine, but can also be done in side lying on the sound side. The patients arm is supported by the therapist with his elbow extended and in external rotation (Bobath 1994).

1. Individual muscle exercise
   In supine lying position
   In side lying
   In sitting
   In standing

2. Functional exercise: The description of functional exercise and the strategies to relearn functional tasks is made in the next chapter on

III b. Activities to restore program control system in the brain:

In the early stage of skill acquisition motor skills are learned and stored as programmed motor activities in the brain. These programmed activities are then available for spontaneous execution and without much voluntary effort. Moreover the program activities are a chain of interconnected, interrelated, organised muscle activities Therefore the program control system is largely responsible for the storing, retrieving and then executing interconnected and interdependent muscle activities. In case of a brain lesion like stroke, this system may either be damaged or disconnected from the periphery; consequently programmed activities are no longer available for spontaneous execution. Individual muscle activities are essential and constitute the baseline activities for the programmed activities; whereas the use of muscle chain exercises and functional exercises constitute the appropriate activities to restore program control system of the brain.

Improve individual muscle function (baseline function of programmed activities) => Use of muscle chain exercise (effective mean in the reacquisition of programmed activities) => Mastering of different functional tasks (effective in restoring program control system in the brain).

Therefore the strategy to restore program control system includes:

- Improve individual muscle activities
- Use of muscle chain exercises
- Relearning functional task

1. Improve individual muscle function:

In the chapter on restoration of feedback control system a detailed description is made to restore individual muscle function.

2. Exercise of the whole muscle chain.

Given that the chained activity of muscle is the part of normal muscle functioning. Initially after birth a child is in a supine position and progressively he/she learns the ability to lay prone, lifting of the head or raising itself on the elbow before developing the capacity of resting on all fours, kneeling and finally standing. In the early stages these activities are used as a mean of skill acquisition. These activities are not only effective in improving muscle function but also in acquisition functional autonomy. That is these exercises help to improve dexterity and strength of individual muscles. Therefore the similar strategies as early skill acquisition can be used in the restoration of program controlled system in the brain. Moreover theses exercises allow hemiplegic subjects to use a wide base and low centre of gravity which is easy to maintain before progression is made to a narrower base with a higher centre of gravity. These exercise are developed by Bobath (1994) who have observed their effectiveness in regaining functional autonomy during her long clinical experience. These exercises according to Bobath (1994) include:

Supine ←=→ Side lying
Supine ←=→ prone lying
Prone lying elbow supported
Prone lying ←=→ four points kneeling
Resting on all fours (four points kneeling)
Moving on all fours (moving forwards and backwards)
Kneeling on all fours ←=→ kneeling
Kneeling (two points kneeling)
Activities in a kneeling position (Walking backwards, forwards and sidewise)
Half kneeling position
Half kneeling ←=→ standing

Turning over from a supine position to lying on the side:
One of the first activities the physiotherapist should work on in treatment is that of turning over to either side (Bobath1992). The following sequences are described by Bobath (1992) to teach turning from supine position to lying on the side:

Turning should begin with the upper part of the body and, in order to do this, the patient must learn to lift the affected arm with the good arm, and to clasp his hand (that is with the fingers interlocked). He should then lift his clasped hands, with the elbows extended to the horizontal position and, if possible, raised above the head. From there he should move his arms first to one side and then to the other. Turning over to the sound side should also be started with the arm and trunk with the hands held clasped. Initially turning has to be done with some help before the subject can learn to do it by themselves.

Turning over from a supine position to lying face down:

Here the subject turns to lying on their side and then to lying prone. Usually turning to the prone position is done in passing by the affected side, where the subject may need the help of their therapist to place her/his arm. The arm supported position can help the subject to improve the stabilisation of the shoulder together with control of the head.

Kneeling on all fours and related activities (four points kneeling):

When the subject kneels on all fours, the weight bearing on the affected arm facilitates the recovery of both the shoulder and elbow stabilisers. The weight on the knee and hip joint also helps to improve the hip stabilisers. Subsequent forwards and backwards movement not only improves the static and dynamic function of the whole upper limb, but it also helps to improve the hips and trunk muscle. However many elderly people may find it to be a very difficult position, especially people with degenerative knee joint problems. Bobath (1992) suggests that treatment in prone kneeling is of limited value in older patients suffering from hemiplegia, many of whom have circulatory problems and cannot tolerate lying prone. Kneeling is often uncomfortable or painful for those who have arthritis and stiff joints, or for those who are very heavy and would probably have difficulty in getting down on the floor and up again even without the complications of hemiplegia.

Kneeling and related activities (two points kneeling):

Kneeling is an important position and very effective in the preparation for walking. In this position the body weight is born by the hip joints, which helps to improve their stabiliser muscles. However, it is often difficult to maintain a full extension of subject's hip in this position, especially that of the affected hip, and there is a tendency for the subject to put less weight on the affected side than on the sound one (Bobath 1994).

It is important that the subject has a good balance in the kneeling position. In the case of a poor balance in this position, some improvement can be obtained through rhythmic stabilisation. Here, the therapist pushes the subject backwards at the level of the shoulder and then stops suddenly so that the subject must try to maintain a kneeling position without falling. A similar exercise can be done laterally, as well as postero-interiorly.

Once good balance in a kneeling position is acquired, the subject can practice walking in this position. Exercises in lateral walking, both on the affected and unaffected side, as well as walking backwards can also be practiced.

2. Relearning of functional tasks

Learning of functional activities constitutes a crucial strategy in the in restoration of program control system in the brain. Although individual muscles are the functional unite of the global task; however the improvement individual muscle function alone may not be effective in restoring program control system in the brain. Carr and Shepherd (2004) state that although the assumption is often made that improved strength will transfer automatically into improved functional ability; however, this may not be case. This statement is based on research over many years by Rutherford (1988), and Morrissery et al (1995), which have demonstrated that exercise effects tend to be specific to task and context. Moreover Hochstenbach and Mulder (1999) suggest that the motor skills have a specific organizational structure; they should not arbitrarily be broken into parts for practice. This organizational structure is largely mediated by program controlled system of the brain. The motor learning literature shows that skills are learned most effectively when they are practiced repeatedly in relation to meaningful goals, incorporating variations in the manner in which they are performed and varying the environment and task (Holden et al 2006, Morris et al 1998, Carr and Shepherd 1998). In addition the program controlled activities are not only the result muscle activities but they are the result of a combined action of sensory, motor and cognitive activities. That is, a combined effect of motor, sensory, and cognitive activities produces an organised kinematic motor activities, which enable one to move around adapt and readjust within their own environment, and improve individual muscle function may not help to improve this kinematic organisation skill.

Moreover a brain lesion impairs the knowledge of the subject's ability to adjust within his/her environment. Mulder (1991) suggests that motor (re)learning, however, is not the relearning of muscle control or movement control but the reacquisition of knowledge and skills of how to move adequately in a continuously changing environment. Moreover the functional tasks constitute relevant information for the brain and therefore they are attended by the brain, and learning is facilitated, In contrast individual muscle activities constitute irrelevant information for the brain and may remain unattended and the objective of skill acquisition may not be achieved. Hochstenbach and Mulder (1999) suggests that better and more efficient remembering and learning will result from keeping the component of a movement sequence that are interrelated and dependent on each other together. Therefore making use of functionally relevant exercise on a repeated basis can be an effective way of reacquiring of this knowledge and eventually of restoring brain function. Relearning of functional activities like getting in and out of the bed, sit to stand, and walking can be the part of functionally relevant exercise and thus an effective mean to restore program control system in the brain. Moreover the skills can be acquired by performing a simple task, consolidate the acquired skill and then progress to more complicated tasks. According to Carr and Shepherd (2004) if rehabilitation is to be effective in optimising functional recovery, an increased emphasis needs to be placed on ways to force the use of the effected limbs through functionally relevant exercise and training. Moreover in the strength training as well as in skill development, repetition is an important aspect in the process of relearning. However a major problem can be encountered while performing different functional tasks, the hemiplegic subject with very weak individual muscle may tend to use compensatory movements in order to overcome the weakness of individual muscle. For example a subject with very weak quadriceps muscle may either walk with a hyperextend knee joint in order to block the knee, or may lean on the sound side to minimise the difficulty to use weak quadriceps. In worse case there may be fall due to inability lock the knee joint resulted from quadriceps weakness. Bobath (1992) argues that in order to get patient walk as soon as possible, the emphasis of treatment is placed on the sound side in compensation of loss of effected side. The author further adds that he is given a tripod on which to lean; which brings the whole weight towards the sound side and makes him use his sound leg for balance and walking. It is therefore critical that a close examination is made of the patient's ability to generate and sustain force as active motor tasks are practised, and that is followed up by exercise and training the specifically targeting the muscles in which weakness is evident and apparently affecting function (Carr and Shepherd 2004).

Moreover mastering of functional tasks has the advantage, which is that once they are learned, they can be repeated several times while performing daily activities, which in turn facilitate the neurogenasis activities of the brain. Given active and repetitive actions are crucial for fostering experience-dependent changes Kempermann et al (1997) and functional reorganisation Lauria et al (1975) in the intact neural circuits of the brain, whereas a bout of exercise in the physiotherapy department two or three times a week may fail to facilitate these kind of changes. Since the objective of relearning different functional tasks is to restore the impaired program controlled activities in the intact neural circuits of the brain, it is therefore essential that the tasks are active and repetitive. Carr and Shepherd (2004) suggest that that training and practice using methods that facilitate motor learning or relearning are essential to the formation of new connections within the remaining brain tissue. An increase of synaptic efficiency in the existing neural circuits in the form of long-term potentiation and the formation of new synapses may be involved in the earlier stages of motor learning (Assuma and Keller 1991). Moreover a large part of an early increase in muscle strength in the able-bodied is due to neural adaptation, including task-specific adaptations to the neural drive, which are both quantitative (an increase of the neural drive to the target muscles) and qualitative (a reduction in co-contraction and an improvement in the coordination among the synergists) Klapp 1975, Schmidt R A (1976), Evarts E V and Tanji (1994), and Schmidt (1982). Therefore it is reasonable to hypothesise that repetitive exercise and training following a stroke may provide a crucial stimulus to creating new or more effective functional connections within the remaining brain tissue Jueptener (1997).

In addition the muscles contract statically or dynamically either to produce a movement at the joint or to ensure the stability of the joint. According to Dolan (1995) muscles will often contract not to cause movement but rather to alter the stress distribution within a bone. For example during the stance phase of the walking cycle, the stabilisers of the hip joint contract statically to transform the tensile stress (bending force) on the neck of the femur into compressive stress (bone is strong in compression and weak in bending). Bone tissue can bare more resistance in compression stress than in bending stress (tensile stress). Moreover bone requires regular compressive force for maintaining its strength, resilience and density. In contrast stress deprivation may facilitate the demineralisation and atrophy of the bone. Muscle weakness and muscle inactivity may not only responsible for bone atrophy but they can also enhance weakness and atrophy of other non-contractile tissues such as ligaments, tendons and joint capsule. Different functional and weight bearing activities are not only effective to reduce stress deprivation on the muscles but also on the bone and other non-contractile tissues and thus prevent their adaptive change.

It is clear that the kinematic organization of motor activities in a functional task is largely mediated by program controlled activities; therefore, relearning of those activities and then integrate them in the tasks of daily living seems an appropriate strategy to restore program control system in the brain. However a task performance is not only a synchronised action of several single muscles, but also it is backed by intact sensory, balance and cognitive activities and these functions can be impaired following a stoke. It is therefore essential that the relearning of functional task as a part of strategy to restore program control system includes:

- Practice and integrate functional activities in daily life tasks.
- Restore balance function
- Restore sensory function
- Relearning of functional tasks taking in to account different cognitive impairments.

Different functional tasks are the result of a combined action of: -Program control activates; - Intact balance function; - Intact sensory function; - and interaction of different cognitive activities.

Functional exercise:
Lying ← → sitting.
Sitting ← → standing.
Walking and turning.
Walking outdoors.

Lying to sitting- getting in and out of bed:

The first movement that has to be learnt is that of turning on both the affected and the unaffected sides. Bobath (1992) describes the following sequence in this exercise; turning should begin with the upper part of the body moving over on the sound side. Turning over on the affected side is easier for the subject than turning on the sound side. Moreover the subject has to learn to move the affected arm and leg to the side. Once the subject is on the sound side, she/he brings their feet out of the bed and sits up by pushing with the sound arm. The subject should also practice moving into a sitting position from lying on the affected side. This can be more difficult and take more time to learn. Repeated practice of the maneuver is essential to restore the function in the intact neural circuits. Moreover the subject thus learns to pay attention to the movements. One way of paying attention to the movements is that the subject should learn to plan and rehearse the sequences before starting. It is important to have a good sitting balance before the subject can practice moving from a lying to a sitting position independently. In the case of poor sitting balance, this sequence can still be practiced, but it needs the constant supervision of the therapist.

A hemiplegic subject who has difficulty to get out of the bed may undertake the following strategy: - Shifting the pelvis toward the centre of the bed so that when turn is completed the body is not too close the edge; - turning the head; - bringing the arms across the body in the direction of rolling; - winging the legs over the edge, - pushing up to sit down, and adjusting postural alignment to sit. The shifting of pelvis involves lifting of the pelvis off the bed and move sidewise. Bending of the legs facilitates lifting of the pelvis, initially subject may be unable to the hemiplegic leg; therefore the lifting of pelvis can be done only by bending the sound leg. Turning on the hemiplegic side is often easier than turning on the sound side; however as the subject lies on his/her hemiplegic arm it would be difficult for the pushing up sequence. In contrast turning on the sound side is difficult given that the subject has to roll his/her hemiplegic arm and trunk on the side and many hemiplegic subjects may find it extremely difficult; however in this position the subject can use his/her sound side to push up, which is much easier (subjects with hemi-negligence will experience extra difficulty turning on the sound side. Therefore, therapist has to try both sides until the subject can perform the task independently. It is important that the subject has good sitting balance before he/she performs this task independently.

Getting into bed:

- Get close to the bed
- Turn round to sit on the bed
- Move the buttocks towards the middle of the bed so that the back of the knees touch the edge of the bed.
- Finally lie on the side and pull the feet onto the bed

Plan and mentally rehearse the sequences before starting.

Standing and sitting down:

Training standing and sitting down following a stroke (STSD) is crucial for regaining independence and mobility and an inability to perform these actions effectively predisposes the individual to a condition of dependence on others for mobility and an increasingly sedentary life style (Carr and Shepherd 2004). In contrast by acquiring independence in STSD many hemiplegic subjects can improve their autonomy of movement. Carr and Shepherd (2004) suggest that every effort should be made to intensive training standing and sitting down, since independence within the real world makes greater use of this ability than that of transferring from one surface to another by pivoting on the non-paretic limb. Physiotherapeutic intervention has the potential to train most patients to recover their independence in this respect.

Before starting to teach subjects how to stand and sit, it is important to ensure that the subject has good sitting balance. Anyone with poor sitting balance will find it extremely difficult to stand up. Similarly poor standing balance can have an inhibiting effect on exercises in standing up and the subject will need constant and close supervision. Moreover the strength of the antigravity muscle of the trunk and the lower limbs are also essential to facilitate practice standing up and sitting down. The length of muscles and other soft tissues also play an essential role in the performance of STSD. It is therefore important that these underlying conditions are taken into account if the subject experiences difficulty in STSD.

According to Carr and Shepherd (2004), though muscle weakness is a limiting factor immediately after a stroke, research has drawn attention to several key mechanical factors that can render practice of this action possible even for a frail patient:

- initial foot position at approximately 75° ankle dorsiflexion as this requires less effort
- adjust seat height in function of the lower limb extensors
- active hip flexion initiated with the trunk vertical (90° to horizontal) to optimize horizontal momentum of the body mass
- no pause between pre-extension and extension phases
- speeding up the action.

The following guidelines for the performance of the exercise in standing up are described by Carr and Shepherd (2004):

Start with upper body in a vertical position with the feet placed back. The subject has to swing his/her upper body forward at the hips and stand up.

- Subject sits on a firm surface
- No arm rests
- Feet on the floor (vary thigh support so that the ankles are dorsiflexed to 75°).
- Adjust the height of the seat to encourage weight to be placed on the affected lower limb and discourage an adaptive redistribution towards the non-paretic limb.

The following guidelines for practicing sitting down are likewise proposed by Carr and Shepherd (2004):

- Patient flexes hips, knees and ankles to lower the body mass towards the seat
- Upper body flexes forward at the hips as the body mass is lowered.
- Weight remains supported over the feet. Nearing the seat, body mass is moved back to enable seat contact.

As noted above, a good sense of balance when sitting and standing, as well as the strength of the lower limb muscles and an optimal length of soft tissue, are important factors in facilitating the performance of STSD. Before practicing STSD the subject can learn to lean forward to touch the floor and sit up again. This improves the strength of the trunk extensors, which can facilitate the performance of standing up and sitting down. However, the important objective is to restore this crucial function in the intact neural circuits so that they are available easily and automatically for execution. This can be achieved by practicing active STSD repeatedly. The subject learns to plan and mentally rehearse the procedure before starting STSD. Paying maximum attention to the movements of the affected limb and trunk is also essential in facilitating experience-dependent change in the intact neural circuits of the brain. Even so, more research is needed using brain imaging control.

Morris (200) suggests the following sequences to facilitate the task of getting out of a chair for people with Parkinson's disease, and the same strategy can be used for stroke patients for relearning of sitting from standing and walking:

- First of all the subject reaches as close as possible to the chair,
- Then turns around so that the chair is behind the subject, and
- Finally bends forward to sit down.
- Plan and mentally rehearse the sequences.

Walking and turning:

Walking: An inability to walk can be one of the most devastating effects of a stroke with severe psychological and physiological consequences. It is important that a maximum effort is made so that hemiplegic subjects can relearn walking with safety. The static and dynamic balance reaction in standing, an adequate force in the individual muscles, a good sensory function of the lower limb muscles constitute important prerequisites for walking. However, most damaging effect of a stroke is that the skill of walking itself, which is stored in the brain, is either destroyed or no more available for execution. Therefore the objective of walking reeducation is to restore the skill of walking in the intact neural circuits of the brain

Gait training should be done from the outset without allowing the subject to use a stick, so that he develops a symmetrical walking pattern with the weight bearing on the affected side. (though the subject should be assisted by the therapist until he has achieved good standing balance and is no longer in danger of falling) (Bobath 1994). Underlying factors like good balance in standing, the strength of the lower limb muscles, deep and superficial sensation and an optimal length of the soft tissues are important for safe and normal walking. Pain in the joint and muscle spasticity may be responsible for a tendency to pathological walking. Therefore relearning walking is a constant process of training and assessment to identify the underlying factors that interfere with the normal process. Reeducation to correct the underlying factors that are responsible for pathological walking and walking reeducation itself can be practiced simultaneously. It is not appropriate to wait until the underlying factors are perfectly in order before starting to walk. In the case of impaired superficial and deep sensation, the subject is taught to use visual sensation to compensate for this loss of somatic sensation. In the case of individual muscle weakness more emphasis in reeducation may be given to the strengthening of individual muscles. Particularly the strength of the knee extensors and hip abductor muscles is important for safe and physiological walking. It is essential to ensure that the subject not use any compensatory movement to overcome this muscle weakness. For example, in the case of weakness of the quadriceps, which is the principal knee extensor, the subject may tend to hyperextend the knee joint in order to ensure stability of the knee. In this condition the weight of the body is born by the soft tissues behind the joint instead of the quadriceps muscle. According to Bobath (1994) the following sequences can be practiced before walking:

- In order to prepare for a reasonably normal gait, balance, stance and weight transfer should be practiced.
- For the swing phase, the patient needs to release his spasticity at the hip, knee and ankle to lift his leg and make a step.
- He also needs to control the extension when putting his leg down to the ground.

Often hemiplegic subjects tend to walk while leaning on the unaffected side and by minimizing the weight bearing on the affected leg. This can produce a limping gait pattern. Therefore to improve the duration of weight bearing on the affected leg, the subject can practice moving forwards and backwards with the unaffected leg while bearing the weight on the affected leg. The important aspect on which the subject needs to concentrate is to lift the unaffected foot slowly and then to place it slowly, while concentrating and feeling the weight bearing on the affected leg.

Carr and Shepherd (2004) suggest the following strategy for walking:
Walking forwards: Starting with the body erect i.e. with the hips extended, the patient steps forwards with the non-affected limb and then the affected limb.

- Initiating the gait with the affected limb in stance sets up the best condition for the subsequent swing phase.
- The goal of the first few steps is for the subject to get a basic locomotive rhythm, while supporting propulsion and balance of the body mass.
- Steady the patient at the upper arm or with the safety belt. Do not interfere with the progression forward.
- Stand at side of the patient or if necessary behind, so as not to impede their vision.
- Encourage subject to step out and take even steps.
- Learn to create a mental map (cognitive map) of the entire trajectory before starting to walk, like going to the other room or the kitchen.
- Use of internally generated instructions or a mental image of taking long steps during walking (Morris and Iansek 1997).

- Attentional strategies such as focusing attention on the key aspects of the gait pattern requiring improvement, while at the same time avoiding the performance of a secondary motor or cognitive task that may compromise safety during the exercise (Morris 2005). However many hemiplegic subjects may have attention disorder and they may not be able to use the function of attention to improve their walking performance. In this case of an impair attention function the subject may have to rely on the automatic aspect of walking, which again can be improved by repeated practice.
- Encourage the subject to walk faster and take longer steps (Carr shepherd 2004). They further suggest that it is difficult to develop an effective locomotive rhythm when walking very slowly. Slow walking disrupts the dynamics of action in both able bodied and disabled subjects and it has been demonstrated that when stroke patients walk at their maximum speed they have a greater symmetry of movement (Wagenaar 1990). A significant relationship has been found between speed and gait parameters (Wagenaar and Beek1992).

Possibility foster neural change to restore program controlled system:

Previously learned movements are generated by program system of the brain. As maintained earlier that the different tasks of daily living activity like getting in and out of the bed, getting in and out of the chair, walking and other more complex activities like running, bicycling, swimming are largely mediated by the program controlled system of the brain. These skills are learned and stored in the brain, which are available to execute easily and quickly. These learned activities are no longer available for automatic execution following a brain damage like cerebro vascular accident. Therefore task specific training can help to restore those functions. Moreover there is evidence that the task specific training has a facilitating effect on the neuroprtection. The objective of different muscle training strategy is to foster the following neural changes:

Experience-dependent changes: The repeated and active performance of different functional tasks may facilitate experience-dependent change in the intact neural circuits, which will help to restore program controlled activities in the brain. It is assumed that repeated and active performance of different tasks will facilitate experience-dependent change in the brain, which in turn will facilitate the restoration of the impaired function, and eventually those functions will be available to execute easily and automatically. Again cognitive function play important role in restoration of those functions, it is therefore important take into account of different cognitive impairment while designing the strategy to restore program controlled system. Especially the attention function plays important role in facilitating different learning activities; therefore, impaired attention function will have hindering effect on relearning of different tasks. However more research is required to identify the kind of activities that facilitate experience-dependent change.

Functional reorganisation: Functional reorganisation in a damaged brain is an important mechanism for the neural recovery, in which impaired brain function is compensated by the other intact areas of the brain. For example the damaged areas that are responsible for the hand function may be taken over by the intact area responsible for shoulder function. Program controlled system is responsible for storing and the automatic retrieving of different learned activities like getting in and out of the bed, sitting from standing and vice versa, walking etc. It is therefore important that the hemiplegic subjects, learns these tasks using attention function, integrate these tasks in daily living activities. From the literature on motor learning it is clear that, as a general rule, the action to be acquired should be practiced in its entirety (task-specific practice), since one component of the action of the action is to a large extent dependent on the preceding components (Carr shepherd 2004). Nudo et al (1996) describe that after repeated training of paralysed hand of the squirrel monkey, the hand representation expanded in to regions formerly occupied by representation of elbow and shoulder. Therefore they concluded that rehabilitative training can shape subsequence reorganisation in the adjacent cortex. According to Carr and Shepherd (2004) representational plasticity of cortical motor maps are provoked by active, repetitive training and practice.

However it appears that repetitive motor activity alone is not sufficient to produce representational plasticity in cortical motor maps (Nudo 2003). Instead, new motor skill acquisition, or motor learning, is a prerequisite factor in driving representational plasticity in the motor cortex (Plautz et al 2000). Relearning of tasks, like getting in and out of a bed, getting in and out of a chair, and walking can be considered as learning of new tasks in hemiplegis subjects. Therefore this relearning or new learning process seems to provoke representational plasticity in the intact neural circuits.

- Facilitate the maturation of newly proliferated neurons: Brain lesion facilitates cell proliferative activities. However stimulation deprivation may facilitate the designation of newly proliferated neurons. In contrast different stimulation in form active task performance and then repeat those tasks during daily activities may facilitate the retention and maturation of the newly proliferated neurons. It is important to facilitate retention and maturation of newly proliferated neurons, because those neurons will in turn be responsible for the restoring different impaired functions.

- Inhibit the competitor neural circuits: Inappropriate activities may reinforce the competitor neural circuits which might have inhibiting effect on functional recovery. Robertson and Murre (2000) suggest that one of the ways in which recovery from brain damage can take place is through the lifting of inhibition over damaged networks by healthy competitor circuits. This can take place either by dampening down the inhibitory competition or by boosting the activation in circuit in the lesioned network. Different intact brain stem and spinal reflex activities might work as a competitor circuits; therefore, it is essential that the therapist observes the subject does not reinforce the spastic pattern during relearning of task performance. However more research is needed with functional magnetic resonance imaging (fMRI) control to indentify the appropriate strategy facilitate neural recovery without reinforcing competitor neural circuits.

Task-specific training facilitates neuroprotection:

Evidences from animal model suggest that pharmacotherapies, learning and exercise may have neuroprotctive influence in neurological disorders (Woodlee and Schallert 2004; Spires and Hannan2005). Woodlee and Schallert (2004) found that the onset of abnormal movements to be prevented or delayed when parkinsonian rats exposed to MPTP (1-methyl-4-phenyl-1,2,3,6-tetrahydropyridine) were trained in an enriched environment. Similarly, rat models of Huntington disease have shown that locomotor training using a treadmill within an enriched environment delays the progression of gait disorders (Spires and Hannan2005). Fisher et al (2002) demonstrated that in medication induced PD rats, treadmill walking for 30 days resulted in walking speed being recovered to the level of nonlesioned animals, along with increased synaptic occupancy of dopamine receptors in the brain. In contrary inactivity may hinder the process of neurogenesis.

However the evidence of the effects of training functional motor task comparing with the effect of training isolated movement is not available (Morris 2000).

It can be concluded that the task specific training may induce experience-dependent change in the intact neural circuit, functional reorganisation, and facilitate the retention and maturation of newly proliferated neuron. Moreover studies have demonstrated that different task specific training has neuroprotective effects. However it is important that different activities should not reinforce the competitor neural circuits and hinder functional recovery. The essential objective of designing rehabilitation strategy is to restore the impaired program controlled system in the brain. More research is required to identify what are the activities that are effective to restore the program controlled system without strengthen the competitor neural circuits.

Conclusion of restoration of program controlled system:

- Kinematic organisations of motor activities in functional tasks are largely mediated by the program controlled system.

- Program controlled activities include different tasks of daily living activities like getting in and out of the bed, getting in and out of a chair, walking.
- Restoration of program controlled system is essential in the rehabilitation of hemiplegic subjects, which in turn enable them to retrieve pre-programmed muscle activities and to execute different tasks easily and spontaneously.
- Strategy of restoration of program controlled system may include exercise of the whole muscle chain and different functional exercises.
- The individual muscle exercise and functional exercises are performed simultaneously in order to restore feedback controlled and program controlled systems; however in case where the subject uses compensatory movement in task performance, more emphasis is placed in the rehabilitation strategy to improve individual muscle function.
- Active and repeated exercises of whole muscle chain, as well as different functional exercises facilitate neuroregenesis activities in the damage brain; like experience dependent change, functional reorganisation, and facilitates maturation of newly proliferated neurons, which in turn can restore the impaired program controlled system in the brain.
- Moreover different task specific training has neuroprotective effects.
- However it is important that different activities to restore program controlled system do not reinforce the competitor neural circuits.

The physical management of uninhibited reflex activities or spasticity:

Bobath (1994) suggests that that the aim of the treatment is to inhibit the released pattern of spasticity so as to help the patient gain control. The restoration of the feedback and the program controlled systems will help to inhibit spasticity, because these two systems exert a modulating and inhibiting influence on the different reflex activities. Muscular spasticity following a stroke is non progressive, though it may take a more prominent role in the event of muscle weakness. In contrast muscular strength may be able to inhibit spasticity or at least minimise its dominating role. Impaired voluntary and automatic activity of muscles is mainly responsible for the presence of dominate reflex muscle activities following stroke. Uninhibited reflex muscle activities have an interfering effect on normal function of the limb. It is therefore important that hemiplegic subjects learn to perform voluntary muscle contraction in a position of spastic inhibition, while at the same time learn to perform functional activities in order to minimise the dominating role of reflex muscle activities.

Many functional exercises are themselves effective in minimising the dominating role of spasticity because they restore the program controlled activities, which have an inhibiting and modulating effect on spasticity. Bobath (1994) suggests that this inhibition cab be obtained by special techniques of patient handling, so as to facilitate a modified disposition of the higher integrated reactions responsible for correction and balance, which is to say of the static-kinetic movement patterns within the normal central postural control mechanism, which provides the automatic background for normal functional skills. To do this, the patient must be helped gradually to gain control over his abnormal postural reflex activity, to bypass the 'short-circuit' into abnormal patterns, and so enable more normal motor functions again to become established. For example, the subject could be placed in a simple lying posture with the limb placed in a position of inhibition, which would facilitate the voluntary activity of the muscles.

A strategy to minimise spasticity:

Muscular spasticity is a hallmark in people with a stroke; the most damaging effect of spasticity is that it interferes in the execution of purposeful movement, while it actually produces uncontrolled and involuntary movements. As discussed above, the muscular spasticity in post stroke hemiplegic patients can be the result of exaggerated spinal reflex activities, uncontrolled postural reaction and the release of postural reflex activities. The abnormal types of postural tone and the stereotypical total motor patterns we see in our patients are the result of disinhibition, i.e. a situation where lower patterns of activity escape from higher inhibitory control (Bobath 1993).

Bobath (1994) suggests that an attempt should therefore be made to change the motor output by giving subjects with hemiplegia more normal sensations of tonus movement and teaching them how to control such movement unaided. The author further suggests that by changing the relative position of parts of the body and limbs when handling a hemiplegic subject, we can change her/his abnormal postural patterns and stop (inhibit) the outflow of excitation. We can at the same time direct the subject's active responses into channels of higher integrated coordination. In this way, spasticity will be reduced through the inhibition of its patterns, while more normal postural reactions and movements are facilitated. However the analysis of motor functional architecture of the central nervous system unveils that the reflex control system is deprived of their inhabiting and modulating effects. This inhibiting and modulating effect is provided by the feedback and program control system. Therefore effort to inhibit spasticity may have little effect for the long term management of spasticity. In contrast, precisely structured stimulations which can restore program and feedback control system, which in turn can effectively exert inhibiting and modulating effect on reflex control system can have long-term effect on reducing spasticity. These stimulations include repeated active movements to improve the voluntary functioning of individual muscles (to restore the feedback control system) and task oriented activities to improve different functional tasks (to restore the program controlled system). It is obvious that spasticity can interfere in the performance of these movements and it is therefore often necessary to place the subject in a position of inhibition in order to facilitate the relearning process. However, simply helping the subject to prevent spasticity will not help to improve program and feedback controlled activities, unless the subject tries to improve these functions actively and by repeated practice. Furthermore muscular spasticity is caused by the release of an abnormal postural reflex mechanism, which results in an exaggerated reflex function at the expense of dynamic postural control (Bobath 1990).

In conclusion, spasticity exerts an interfering role in the execution of various movements and functional tasks. Inhibiting spasticity may facilitate the performance of these different tasks. However the release of spastic pattern is mainly due to the absence of the inhibiting and modulating effects on the reflex controlled activities, from the program and feedback controlled activities. Therefore it is reasonable to improve program and feedback controlled activities so that they can exert an inhibiting and modulating effect the involuntary and reflex muscles. In other words it is important to learn different exercises to improve voluntary muscle activities (restore the feedback control system), as well as to improve spontaneous muscle function (restore the program controlled system). It is obvious though that the different exercises need to be practiced in a position of inhibition to start with, at least until the subjects have sufficient control over these movements, in order to avoid the interfering effects of spasticity on movements concerned. Unfortunately only minimising uninhibited reflex activities may not be able to restore program control and feedback control system in the brain and without their restoration hemiplegic subjects will continue experience difficulty to produce purposeful movements and task performance. Moreover programme and feedback control system impairments are not only responsible for the difficulty to perform purposeful movements but also they are responsible to perpetuate inhibited reflex activities and their restoration can only be achieved by providing precisely shaped stimulation received by the brain. More data is needed, which are validated with brain's electromagnetic resonance image, in order to identify what are the precisely shaped stimulation to restore program and feedback control system in the brain. It can be concluded that the dominant reflex activities are the result of impaired feedback and program control system of the brain, it is therefore crucial to restore these two systems in order to minimise the dominating effect of reflex activities or spasticity.

VI
Restore Sensory Function

The function of sensation in both its regulatory and adaptive modes (Gordon 2000) serves both to guide movement during execution and to correct it so as to improve the next attempt. Sensory impairment is common following a stroke and, if present, this related problem may add considerably to a patient's difficulties and adversely influence their chances of recovery from functional disability. Thus the restoration of sensory function constitutes an essential aspect in stroke rehabilitation. The various sensory functions include the superficial and profound sensation of the body, as well as the visual and auditory awareness. However it is important to distinguish between the presence of cognitive dysfunction and sensory impairment. For example, hemineglect is a dysfunction of hemicorps and hemispace, which can display similar symptoms in failing attention and perception as sensory impairment. It is therefore essential to identify the type of sensory impairment present and distinguish these sensory problems from different cognitive problems. The following discussion examines the consequences of sensory dysfunction in hemiplegic subjects, after which some strategies for the restoration of this sensory function will be discussed.

Consequences of impaired sensory function:

Partial or complete loss of discrete sensation (tactile or proprioceptive) and perceptual-cognitive disorders (visiospatial impairments, inattention) impacts upon motor behaviour to varying degrees (Carre and Shepherd 2004). Loss of discrete sensation represents a failure of impulses from the various sense organs of skin, joints, muscles, ears, eyes and mouth to reach the relevant areas of the brain (Carey 1995). The sensory stimuli include exterioception (visual and auditory sensation) and interioception (superficial profound sensation and joint position sense). It is therefore essential to identify the exact nature of the sensory impairment before starting to repair its functionality.

Feedback controlled movements are largely dependent on sensory feedback. Movements are performed in response to sensory stimuli which act upon the central nervous system from the outside world (Bobath 1990). Poor sensory feedback from the lower limb joints may be responsible for joint instability or in extreme cases sensory ataxia. The instability of the joint and sensory ataxia can be further aggravated as a result of impaired superficial sensations. This sensory ataxia can impede walking and increase the likelihood of falling. The effect of instability or ataxia due to impaired superficial and deep sensation may be compensated by using visual sensation. It is known that vision provides powerful intrinsic feedback concerning environmental conditions and exterioceptive information for determining the individual's relative position within the environment (Lee and Aronson 1974). However ataxia resulting from the lesion of the cerebellum may not always be reduced through visual control. The most devastating effect of sensory impairment is its interfering effect on the neural recovery. The sensory messages are integrated at various levels of the central nervous system and a coordinated response is produced in step with the demands of the environment (Bobath 1990). In the absence of such sensory stimulation, the central nervous system will be deprived of this environmental feedback, which can in turn hinder neural recovery. Different strategies must thus be envisaged with a view to restoring this sensory function.

Some possible strategies to restore impaired sensory function:

An essential aspect of hemiplegic rehabilitation is to restore sensory function and when necessary teach the subjects to adapt to their sensory impairment. Yekutiel and Guttman (1993) suggest that it is essential to incorporate both sensory and motor training into rehabilitation in a systematic way. Impaired sensory functions can prove a serious impediment to the performance of a wide range of tasks, even though its restoration does not necessarily lead to an improvement in this respect. Whether or not an improvement in sensory perception leads to more effective functional performance is yet unclear (Carr and Shepherd 2004). In this context Carey et al (1993), Yekutiel and Guttman (1993) suggest that specific training in somatosensory perception can be effective. The execution of many different functional tasks like sitting and standing up are not alone effective for muscle recovery but can also play an important role in the restoration of the impaired sensory functions within the body.

It is likely that task-specific practices impact on sensory discrimination, since the nervous system is selective in utilising those sensory inputs most relevant to any particular action (Carre and Shepherd 2004). The authors further suggest that the practice of meaningful tasks and specific exercises may give the damaged system the opportunity to regain the ability to recognise, select and use those sensory inputs that are relevant to the action being performed. For example, practice in standing up and sitting down provides an opportunity to make use of the input from tactile receptors in the soles of the feet. Hemiplegic subjects should pay full attention to such task performance, which can have a facilitating effect on sensory recovery. This training can involve actually cueing the individual about the sensory information required for any specific task (Carr and Shepherd 2004).

Useful challenges involving the hand as a sense organ can sometimes be addressed by focusing the patient's attention on the form of sensory input and its relationship to the task in question (Yekutiel and Guttman 1993). Hyvarinen et al (1980) have also found in an animal study that focusing attention increases the responsiveness of cells in the sensory motor cortex. Therefore encouraging patients to pay maximum attention to the relevant sensory cues (e.g. visual and tactile, as well as those involving muscle force) by setting up an environment appropriate to the task and providing verbal and visual feedback as re-enforcers, may not only affect motor performance but may also improve sensory awareness (Carr and Shepherd 2004).

The sensory training proposed by Yekutiel and Guttman (1993), which involved 45-minute sessions three times a week for six weeks, was based on the following principals:

- The nature and extent of sensory loss must first be explored with the patient.
- Emphasis should be placed on sensory tasks the patient can perform and each session ought to start and end with these.
- Tasks of interest to the patient are to be chosen.
- Use can be made of vision and the non-paretic hand to teach tactics of perception.
- Frequent change of tasks with intermittent periods of rest may help to maximise the patient's concentration.

Progressive functional exercise with and without visual control:

The execution of functional tasks in the progressive position, which are designed to recover muscle function, can help to restore both deep and superficial sensory functions when performed in alternation with and without visual control.

Example of a functional task in the progressive position:

- While walking on all fours the subject is asked to turn her/his head to control the movement of the paralytic arm and leg and progression is made when the subject can perform these same tasks without turning the head but simply keeping their eyes open and then finally the same task is performed with the eyes closed (it should be noted that this four point kneeling and walking can be extremely difficult for many elderly people and those suffering from osteoarthritis of the knee and in this case such an exercise would only have a limited value).
- Walking in a kneeling position using the same strategy of adapting direct visual control (first turning the head towards

the paralytic lower limb followed by an indirect visual control by keeping the eyes open and then finally with the eyes closed). Again this type of exercise can be extremely difficult for many elderly people and people with osteoarthritis of the knee.
- Walking with direct visual control by turning the eyes toward the paralytic lower limb, then with indirect visual control, and then finally with the eyes closed.

Conclusion:

Sensory function is important to regulate and adapt different movements in a constantly changing environment. Many hemiplegics have severe sensory impairment, which has an adverse effect on motor behaviour, as well as impeding any long term functional recovery. This sensory function, however, has to be considered from different aspects, which include interioception (superficial and profound sensation), and proprioception (joint position awareness), exterioception (visual and auditory perception). Impairment can affect either an isolated sensory function or several different functions at the same time and it is therefore important to identify the exact nature of the impairment. Feedback controlled movements are largely dependent on sensory feedback. Impaired deep sensation can result in sensory ataxia, which can be minimised by using visual control of the limb. The most damaging effect of impaired sensory function is that it deprives the brain of varied stimulation, which in turn can hamper the neural recovery.

As in the case of motor rehabilitation it is essential to adapt different strategies to achieve the restoration of sensory function. The execution of specific tasks like sitting and standing up appears to be effective in this respect. Concentrating the attention on the task being performed can also help in fostering neural recovery and the restoration of sensory functions. In addition progressive functional exercise first using and then without visual control is also effective in restoring deep and superficial sensory functions.

Summary of sensory rehabilitation:

> 1. Sensory function is essential to guide and adapt movements during their execution.
> - Hemiplegic subjects can have sensory impairment, which can have an adverse effect on functional recovery.
> - Feedback controlled movements are largely dependent on sensory function and thus neural recovery will be hindered where the damaged brain is deprived of essential sensory stimulation.
> - Different aspects of sensory function include exterioception (visual and auditory sensation) and interioception (superficial and profound sensation, as well as awareness of joint position).
> - Since both individual and grouped sensory functions can be impaired, it is important to begin by identifying the exact nature and scope of the impairment.
> 2. Strategies to restore sensory function include:
> Functional exercises with maximum attention paid to the task performance
> Functional exercises with and without visual control.

VII

Restore Balance Function in People Following a Stroke

Balance reaction enables one to maintain an upright position and perform different activities from that position. According to Berg (1989) balance can be viewed as prerequisite to functional activities as it forms the baseline requirement necessary to carry out many of the activities of daily living. Hence balance can be defined as the body's ability to readjust the postural instability caused during voluntary movement and as a result of reaction to an external disturbance. The ability to balance in an upright position is the power, which enables an individual to maintain or regain the centre of mass over the base of support when faced with altered environmental conditions. This power is provided by a combined effect of sensory, motor and cognitive activities. Moreover MacKinnon and Winter (1993) suggests that balance involves the regulation of the movement of linked body segments over the supporting joints and the base of support. That is, it is the ability to balance the body mass relative to the base of support, enabling us to perform everyday actions effectively and efficiently (Carr and Shepherd 2004). In contrast, an impaired balance reaction can severely hinder the capacity to perform activities in an upright position. Many hemiplegic subjects can have balance impairment, which can severely hinder their ability to regain functional autonomy. It is therefore essential to identify the presence of balance impairment in hemiplegic subject and then undertake measures appropriate to its restoration. The following discussion will examine the consequences of balance impairment, the underlying factors responsible for balance impairment in hemiplegic subjects and finally some strategies reeducate balance impairment is discussed.

The consequences of balance dysfunction in hemiplegic subjects:

Balance dysfunction, particularly when standing, is a devastating sequel of stroke since the ability to balance the body mass over the base of support under different task and environmental conditions is one of the most crucial motor control factors in daily life (Carr and Shepherd 2004). It follows that hemiplegic subjects with impaired standing balance will be confronted with severe difficulty if not the impossibility in standing upright. Not only standing balance but also the sitting balance may be impaired in a severe stroke. In case of an impaired sitting balance hemiplegic subjects will experience difficulty in performing tasks from a sitting position. Such difficulties include that of getting in and out bed or moving from the bed to a chair or a chair to a couch.

A positive "pull test", which consists of a sudden and unexpected sensation of pulling from behind thus provoking balance loss or disturbance, even when they are able to maintain a standing position, is an indication of having balance impairment. Whereas normal individuals react in a "pull test" by dorsiflexing their ankles, lifting the arms forward and in some cases flexing forward at the hips and then stepping backwards, in the case of an impaired balance, these reactions are absent or diminished in amplitude. In the context of the positive pull test hemiplegic subjects may find it difficult to balance body mass over the base of support under different task and environmental conditions. Consequently they may encounter difficulty in walking or performing other tasks from a standing position.

Studies using support-surface perturbation have identified several distinguishing postural abnormalities in people with impaired balance function (Rogers 1996, and Bloem et al 2001):

- Exaggerated automatic postural responses, in particular an enlarged "medium latency" stretch response of the lower leg muscles.

- Inability to modulate the response magnitude to different postural demands.
- Delayed initiation or reduced scaling of voluntary postural responses.
- Abnormal execution of compensatory stepping movements.

These abnormalities can make it difficult to walk or perform other functional tasks from a standing position. Moreover the incidences of falling increase in hemiplegic subjects with an impaired balance reaction. Carr and Shepherd (2003) state that the likelihood of falling increases in the weak and frail, or in the presence of an impairment affecting the neuromuscular or sensory systems, since under these conditions complex actions can no longer be performed effectively. Tinitti et al (1988) and Nevitt et al (1989) have also noted that falls are the main cause of morbidity in otherwise normal elderly subjects, who thus suffer a loss of autonomy and consequent institutionalisation. Many stroke subjects fall into this category with an already present balance impairment, which may be further aggravated as a result. It is therefore essential to identify the balance impairment in hemiplegic subjects and take all necessary measures to restore their balance function.

Underlying factors responsible for the impaired balance function in Hemiplegic subjects:

1. Impaired program controlled activity of muscles: Hemiplegic subjects with impaired program controlled activity will experience the inability regain body mass relative to the base of support in case of sudden change of position. This is mainly due to a failure in kinematic organization in muscle activities.
2. Impair feedback controlled activities of muscles: Carr and Shepherd (2004) suggest that in the wake of a stroke, patients with muscle weakness and poor control may lack effective anticipatory and ongoing reactive postural adjustments.
3. Spasticity: Spasticity produces abnormal activities of muscle and therefore the complex action required for balancing and

maintaining upright position can no longer be performed effectively.

4. Impairment of function of the cerebellum: The sensory input about body position during activities is conveyed to the cerebellum via sensory association cortex of the brain, cerebellum in turn sends afferent impulse via premotor and motor cortex to produce static or dynamic activities of muscles to produce coordinated activities of the limb and the trunk. Cerebellum with its connection with the vestibular apparatus, which helps to regulates balance in upright position (Chez and Fahn 1985). Input from the cerebral cortex is conveyed to the cerebellum through pontine nuclei. A break down in connection between cerebral cortex and cerebellum as well as cerebrospinal connection can result in an instability of the limbs and the trunk in maintaining of upright position and during walking (cerebellar ataxia).

5. Impaired sensory function: Sensory functions include both superficial and deep bodily sensation, as well as positional awareness (proprioception), and visual perception (extrioception). These sensory functions play an important role in maintaining the upright position of the body and in performing function from that position. Winter et al (1990) suggest that redundancy in the sensory system provides for some degree of compensation. For example in the case of an impaired superficial and deep sensation, visual sensation can be used to compensate this loss. Moreover sensory input from the vestibular apparatus plays an important role in maintaining the upright position of the body.

6. Impaired cognitive function: Some cognitive functions also play an important role in maintaining upright position and during performance of complex activities from that position. Hemineglect or hemi-inattention, which is a disorder affecting the selection and structuring of input received by the affected hemi corps, can severely disrupt the subject's ability to maintain an upright position, even that of sitting. Moreover an impaired attention function may hinder a subject's ability to prioritise muscle activity in a synchronised manner during

the performance of a dynamic task. It has been observed that falls are common in elderly people with attention dysfunction. Dietrich and Brandt (1992) suggest that the additional factors likely to impact on stability include abnormal perception of verticality and other disorders of visuospatial perception. Attention and visuospatial perception can therefore be considered as the baseline skill enabling one to perform functional tasks effectively. In contrast there impairment can not only have a hindering effect in attaining functional autonomy but also the prevalence of falls is high in people with cognitive impairment. It is therefore essential to identify the presence of cognitive impairment improve the patient's capacity to support their body mass over the paretic lower limbs, as well as voluntary movements of the body mass from one lower limb or position to another, and responding rapidly to predicted and unpredicted threats to balance.

Possible strategies to restore balance function:

Balance results from the coordinated action of different sensory, cognitive functions, together with voluntary and involuntary muscle activity (program controlled, feedback controlled and reflex muscle activities).

Carr and Shepherd (2004) suggest that ongoing postural adjustment involves:

- Supporting body mass over the paretic lower limb
- Moving the body mass from one lower limb to the other or one position to another.
- Responding rapidly to any threat to balance.

Various strategies to improve balance function may include:
- Restoration of program control system
- Restoration of feedback control system
- Restore sensory impairment and adapt activities according to different sensory losses.

- Restore cognitive function, identify interfering effects of cognitive function, and plan rehabilitation strategies taking in to account different cognitive impairments

Finally each subject should be prepared to maintain a sitting and standing position, while at the same time working to improve stability in different positions by moving from the most stable state to a least stable state. Since the restoration of the muscle, sensory and cognitive functions have already been discussed in other chapters, so the following discussion will examine the techniques to promote stability in sitting and in standing position.

Restore balance function in sitting position:

People with severe hemiplegia may not be able to keep themselves in a sitting position. The ability thus, to maintain a sense of balance while reaching for objects both within and beyond arm's length is critical for independent living (Carr and Shepherd 2004). People with poor sitting balance will be unable to perform other simple task like getting out of the bed or moving from the bed to a wheel chair independently. It follows that re-establishing sitting balance should be one of the first priorities of rehabilitation following a stroke. Carr and Shepherd (2004) suggest that re-establishing sitting balance early is critical since it impacts positively on many functions.

With the subject sitting on a firm surface, the therapist in front should apply a rhythmic stabilization both from the rear and sides, which consists of the application and subsequent rapid release of a firm pressure at shoulder level obliging the patient to try and maintain the sitting position without losing balance. This rhythmic stabilization technique improves subject's static balance. It is also important that the subjects learn to improve their dynamic sitting balance while moving and acting in this position. This requires the subjects to learn certain movements of the head and trunk, as well as practicing the action of reaching while seated.

Head and trunk movements in sitting position:

Carr and Shepherd (2004) have described the following exercises to improve head and trunk movement in the sitting position:

- Sitting on firm surface, hands on lap, feet and knees approximately 15cm apart, feet on floor.
- Turning head and trunk to look over the shoulder, turning to the mid position and then repeating to other side.
- Looking up at the ceiling and returning to upright position.

Reaching action:

Carr and Shepherd (2004) have described the following exercises to improve stability while reaching from the sitting position:

- Sitting, reaching to touch objects with the paretic hand: (forward flexing at the hips), sideways (both sides), backwards, returning to the mid position.
- Reaching to pick up objects from the floor, forward and sideways, one hand and two hands.

Standing balance: Hemiplegic subjects with poor standing balance will be unable to walk with security. It is therefore essential that the subject achieve a good standing balance before she/he starts walking independently. Learning to balance, while standing, requires the opportunity to practice voluntary actions in this position from early on in the acute stage. As with sitting balance, different strategies to improve standing balance include:

- Reactivation of the voluntary and involuntary functions of lower limb and trunk muscles (program and feedback controlled systems).
- Restoration of the sensory functions.
- Identifying cognitive dysfunction and undertake appropriate measures to minimize their hindering effects on balance function.

- Preparation of hemiplegic subjects to maintain the standing position and restore the capacity to perform functions in this position with security.

Restore balance in standing position (Carr and Shepherd 2004 have described the following exercises to improve stability):

- Standing with feet a few cm apart, first look up at the ceiling and then return to a normal upright position.
- Starting from the same position, first turn the head and body mass and look behind before returning to the point of departure and repeat the exercise on the other side.
- From a standing position reach forwards, sideways (both sides) and then backwards to touch an object first with one hand and then with both. This can be done with differing objects in a variety of circumstances. The object should be placed beyond arm's length so challenging the patient to extent the limit of stability and return.
- Single leg support: This exercise can be practiced while stepping forward and placing the weight on the non-paretic limb, though extra care is required especially where trying this single leg support on the paretic limb, where in certain cases the neck of the femur can be subjected to tensile stress because of insufficient glutinous medias muscle which contracts to convert the tensile force in the neck of the femur into a compressive force thus rendering it stronger. That is to say, like other bone the neck of the femur can bear more weight when subjected to compressive rather than tensile (bending) stress. It follows that the likelihood of a fracture in the neck of the femur may increase, when as a result of weak gluteus medias muscle it may be unable to transform tensile stress on the neck into compressive stress. Given the compressive stress on the neck of femur is transformed in to compressive stress as result of effective contraction of the gluteus medias muscle.
- Walking sideways with hand(s) on the wall.

- Picking up objects: Starting from a standing position first lower the body mass to pick up or touch an object by moving forwards, sideways, backwards and then return.

N.B. Hemiplegic subjects need to have sufficient stability in the standing position before practicing single leg support or walking sideways and picking up objects.

Develop stability progressively by moving from simple to complex position:

Waddington (1989) suggests that as a general principal balance is developed progressively by moving from the most to the least stable position, as for example from Forearm Support or Prone Lying to Standing with the aid of sticks. Moreover these exercises enable the subject to master a simple position with a low centre of gravity and a wide base before progressing to an unstable position. However there is no fixed rule that the subject has to master this simple position before progressing to a more difficult one. The therapist may help the subject to try the most difficult position even when she/he has not already mastered the more simple one to which they can come back later. According to Waddington (1989) the following positions may be practiced, all of which enable hemiplegic subjects to gain experience with an easy position before progressing to more difficult ones and thus helping them to improve their sense of balance. In each of these positions the therapist can decide to apply the Rhythmic Stabilisation technique. A gradual increase of alternative resistance is used to build up a co-contraction, i.e. the Rhythmic Stabilisation and the selection of components needed to maintain a particular position can be chosen from the head, shoulder, pelvis or knees (Waddington 1989). In this way the hemiplegic subject can perform different activities in each position.

The different progressive positions proposed by Waddington (1989) are as follows:

- Lying prone with forearm support
- Kneeling with forearm support

- Kneeling on all fours
- Kneeling
- Half Kneeling
- Standing
- Standing on one leg

The main purpose is to learn to adjust the muscle tone to maintain the above positions and then to adjust the posture to maintain or regain the position (the activities in these positions are described in the chapter on restoration of program controlled activities).

Conclusion: Balance reaction is an important function enabling us to maintain an upright position. An impaired balance function may severely hinder a person's ability to perform different tasks in an upright position. This sense of balance may be impaired as a result of a stroke, when the subject is no longer able to keep standing and perform different functions in this position. In the case of a severe stroke the sitting balance may also be affected. A poor sense of sitting balance can prevent a person from performing such mundane tasks as getting in and out of the bed or moving from the bed to a chair. This balance impairment is the result of a combination of dysfunctions, which include both voluntary and involuntary muscle dysfunction, as well as sensory and cognitive impairment. This is then responsible for the lack of an effective system of pro- and reactive postural adjustment.

It is thus essential that hemiplegic subjects improve their sitting and standing balance. Strategies to improve both sitting and standing balance include:

- Restoration of both the program and feedback controlled activities of the muscles of the lower limbs and trunk.
- Restoration of the profound and superficial sensory functions, though the subject can also use visual sensation where these sensory functions are severely impaired.
- Identification of the different forms of cognitive impairment and work to minimize their adverse effects.
- Preparation to improve stability in the sitting and standing positions.

In addition Waddington (1989) suggests that the sense of balance can be improved by teaching people to exercise in different positions, starting in a simple position with a low centre of gravity and wide base and then progressing to a higher centre of gravity or a narrow base. That is to say, the subject should try to progress from a position lying down using forearm support to that of standing upright. Here the Rhythmic Stabilization technique can be applied for each different component of the body and in each position. The subjects can also learn to perform activities in each of these positions.

Summary of balance rehabilitation in people following a stroke:

- Balance is an important function enabling one to maintain an upright position and perform tasks from that position.
- In stroke both the sitting and standing balance can be impaired, which depend on the severity of brain lesion.

Balance impairment following a stroke results from:
- Impaired program controlled activities of muscles
- Impaired feedback controlled activities of muscles
- Spasticity
- Impaired cerebral activities
- Sensory impairment
- Cognitive impairment.
- For this reason any strategy to improve the sense of balance should include the restoration of these three functions (motor, sensory and cognitive function) and then prepare the subject to undertake activities from both a sitting and a standing position.
  Waddington (1989) suggests strategy which includes a progressive development by moving from the most stable to the least stable position.
- In addition the rhythmic stabilization technique can be used in each position for the performance of activities to restore the sense of balance.

VII

Different Cognitive Dysfunctions in Hemiplegic Subjects and their Repercussion in Attaining Functional Recovery

Cognitive dysfunction in people after a stroke:

A stroke is not a 'bundle' of sensori-motor problems but an extremely complex breakdown of many neural systems, leading to motor as well as perceptual, cognitive, and behavioural problems (Hochstenbach and Mulder 1999). Several studies have indicated that cognitive consequences play an important role in stroke rehabilitation and significantly affect the ability of a patient to adjust to neural damage (Feigenson et al 1977; Allen 1984; Novack et al 1987; Sundet et al 1988; Tatenmichi et al 1994). Rehabilitation of hemiplegics is relearning of movements and reacquisition of functional autonomy and different cognitive impairment can have a hindering effect on this relearning process. Mulder (1993) suggests that motor (re) learning is not the learning to control muscles or movement but rather the reacquisition of the knowledge and skills necessary to function adequately in a constantly changing environment. Different cognitive functions play a vital role in this process of knowledge and skill acquisition.

The most damaging effect of impaired cognitive function is that it hinders the process of neuronal recovery. Racanzone et al (1993) state that experience-dependent plastic reorganisation depends on attention being paid by the recipient to the stimulation responsible for such changes. The attention systems of the brain might therefore have a privileged role in functional recovery following brain damage (Robertson et al 1997). Various forms of cognitive impairment can deprive the damaged brain of the necessary stimulation needed for neural reorganisation following a stroke. There is ample evidence that, particularly in the early phases of this learning process, cognitive factors play a crucial role (Proctor and Dutta 1995). Certain cognitive functions play a vital role in enabling one to maintain independent and purposeful life. Therefore the repercussions of different cognitive dysfunctions can include:

- An interfering effect on relearning of motor function.
- Some cognitive dysfunctions hinder the process of neural recovery.
- And finally cognitive function like executive function plays a crucial role in leading an independent and purposeful life.

Hemiplegic subjects can present with different types of cognitive dysfunction, and each dysfunction has its own adverse effect in relearning of motor function and in attaining functional autonomy. Therefore it is crucial in a stroke rehabilitation program to identify the type of cognitive impairment and adjust rehabilitation strategies accordingly. The following discussion integrates some of the research finding to provide the insights of the consequences of cognitive dysfunctions on motor learning process and then some common cognitive dysfunctions that can exist in people after a stroke are also discussed. The discussion limits to five common cognitive impairments, which are the executive problem, memory disorder, disorder in the selection and evaluation of input (hemi-neglect), appraxia and attention disorder.

Role of cognitive function in learning motor function:

Memory as well as learning is context dependent, meaning that an important factor in the retention of motor skills is the relationship between the context of practice and the context of application.

The relevance and rehearsing of information are the two essential ingredients constitute the prerequisite for learning. Similarly Attention and memory are two main cognitive functions mediate in learning and then transform learning into knowledge. Hochchstenbach and Mulder (1999) suggest that learning skills is totally dependent on memory, on the capacity to hold information about ongoing actions and event. Therefore learning motor function requires attention of the information and then storage of information. The storing process is mediated by two different memory functions, which are short-term memory (STM) and long-term memory (LTM). Initially the attention function picks up the information from the environment, information is stored in a STM buffer, which is also working memory, and this forms a transient memory process which lasts from about a few seconds up to few minutes (Magill 1993). As, the storage of short term memory is transient, so to use the information in the future it is necessary the selected information is transferred LTM store (Hochchstenbach and Mulder 1999). Relevance of information is essential to be attended. In contrast the irrelevant information may remain unattended, which neither will reach in the short term nor in the long term memory. Moreover Hochchstenbach and Mulder (1999) state that since motor skills have a specific organizational structure, they should not be arbitrarily broken into parts for practice; better and more efficient remembering and learning will result from keeping the components of a movement sequence that are interrelated and dependent on each other together. In other words the functional tasks constitute the relevant information for the brain while individual movements do not. Therefore functional tasks are better remembered than isolated movements. Furthermore the brain's structure is organized as such that it can store and retrieve the whole component of movement within a functional task. In contrast the individual movements are the result of conscious voluntary effort and may be considered as irrelevant information by the brain. However in the presence of a very weak component of movement within a task, the task performance can be difficult, in which case strengthening of individual muscle is necessary.

In addition two major types of knowledge are stored in LTM, which are mediated by two different brain systems. The first one, the implicit or procedural memory, deals with knowledge on how to perform activities. The second is called explicit or declarative memory, and involves factual knowledge (Squire et al 1993). So, selection of the most adequate motor action involves the explicit memory system, whereas the performance of the action involves the implicit memory system (Hochchstenbach and Mulder 1999). It is clear then that in the process of relearning of motor function and reacquisition of functional autonomy, the interaction of different cognitive function is essential. Therefore it is crucial in stroke rehabilitation not only to identify the presence of cognitive dysfunction but also to adapt different relearning strategies accordingly.

1. Executive function:

An impairment of the executive function can have the most debilitating effects on hemiplegic subjects striving to recover their independence in the activities of daily life. Lezak (1995) defines executive functions as those capacities that enable a person to engage successfully in independent, purposeful and self-serving behaviour. Executive function enables one to conduct planned organised activities of daily living. Hochestbach and Mulder (1999) affirm that for these patients it can be extremely difficult to exercise control over their own lives with the result that they are mostly dependent on external structures, routines and other people, which provides little room for flexibility. They further argue that the extent of dependency varies according to the seriousness of the dysexecutive syndrome and the presence of other cognitive and emotional disorders. Lezak (1992) affirms that an impairment of the executive function may compromise a person's capacity to maintain an independent, constructive, self-serving and socially productive life no matter how well they can see and hear, walk and talk or perform in other tests. Subjects with this disorder of the executive function would be unable to plan and then take the necessary actions to perform the essential activities of daily life.

Lezak (1992) conducted an experiment in building with tinker-toys on a group of thirty-five unselected patients (17 were classified dependent and 18 were classified non-dependent), as well as a group of ten normal control subjects. They were evaluated according to the number of pieces (*np*) used and also the complexity of the tasks performed (*comp*). Results showed that the dependent patients used less than 23 pieces, those were not dependent used more than 23 pieces, whereas half of the control group used all 50 pieces. According to Lezak (1992) the high scoring constructions involved a number of executive functions, including the ability to formulate a goal and plan, as well as initiating and carrying out complex activities in pursuit of that goal. It can therefore be assumed that the subjects with a low score were dependent and suffered from a disorder of the executive function. It must be said that in this research the exact nature of neurological deficit of the participants was not specified. Nor does it serve to highlight any of the possible compensatory measures that could be undertaken to enable patients to cope with their executive problem. Certainly more research is needed to identify the number of hemiplegic subjects with executive dysfunction and discover the possible measures that can help them to overcome this problem.

It can be concluded that people with executive dysfunction will experience difficulty in planning, taking initiatives and performing many of the activities involved in looking after themselves on a daily basis. Depending on the severity of this executive dysfunction and the presence of other problems hemiplegic subjects may thus be dependent on others for many of the essential tasks of daily life. This increasingly passive mode of living may then in turn severely limit the benefits of other neuro-remodelling activities.

2. Aprexia:

Hemiplegic subjects affected by aprexia are generally dependent on others for many of the activities of daily life, though this depends on the severity of the aprexia and the presence of associated dysfunctions. According to De Rengi (1999) and Goldberg (1995) limb aprexia is characterised by the inability to imitate action, to mimic tool use or to perform gesture in response to verbal command. According to Ietswaart et al (2001) aprexia may be described as the dissociation of movements programmed de *novo* with movements copied from a stored representation. Hemiplegic subjects with aprexia will experience difficulty in using many of the tools of daily life, such as a fork, a spoon or a tooth brush; they will have particular difficulty in learning to use a wheel chair or in relearning functional tasks like walking or moving from one place to another. It is crucial to understand that such difficulties in mimicking the use of tools or performing other gestures in response to verbal command are not linked to a memory dysfunction.

Hailman (1979) states that apraxia results from the 'destruction' of the spatiotemporal representation of learned movements. Thus even when the voluntary motor system remains intact; subjects with apraxia would be unable to perform purposeful motor activities. It is interesting that apraxia is not limited to previously learned motor acts and can also be observed in copying novel movements with no meaning (Goldenberg 1993). Patients with apraxia may not be able to perform activities like washing themselves, opening the door or dressing and undressing, mainly because the stored perceptual information of these learned movements are no longer available to the frontal system. During re-education for the performance of different functional tasks like moving from a standing to a sitting position, many therapists use a demonstrative approach, modelling the action to assist the subject in getting an idea of its spatial and temporal features, the 'shape' or topology of the movement (Carr and Shepherd 2004). Hemiplegic patients with aprexia will either be unable or at least experience difficulty in imitating these gestures. They will experience extra difficulty in performing new activities or using new instruments, like manoeuvring a wheel chair. Here it is clear that the standard therapeutic activities would fail to provide appropriate stimulation necessary for neural recovery. However many hemiplegic subjects can overcome the difficulties linked to aprexia by recreating the necessary perceptual information through the intact sensory and motor functions. It is for this reason that the severity of the impact of aprexia is often dependent on the presence of associated cognitive and sensoriomotor dysfunctions.

Ietswaart et al (2001) conducted research shortly after a stroke on ten right-handed hemiplegic subjects suffering from an ischemic infarct of the left cerebral hemisphere; in this study the Goldenberg (Goldenberg 1993) ten meaningless gesture test (this test requires patients to imitate a series of meaningless gestures) was performed with the ipsilateral hand in order to evaluate aprexia. These same patients were then tested again on average 108 days after the stroke (standard deviation = 65). Their performances were compared with those of ten control subjects matched for sex and age. The results of this study provide no evidence that apraxic patients are disproportionately affected in movements based on stored representation. The authors concluded that apraxic patients might be deficient in imitation because their transformation of the visual model to the motor act is compromised. According to this model aprexia falls into the category of sensory impairment rather than being considered as a cognitive problem. However Ietswaart et al (2001) suggest that attention should be paid to the complex interactions involved in transforming sensory information into purposeful acts. Milner (1998) likewise affirms that the perceptual system can provide a conscious awareness of its products in normal individuals by virtue of the fact that it interacts with a stored base of knowledge and awareness of context, which are key features of clinical aprexia. The data obtained from this research showed that all ten patients had a score ranging from 2 – 12 out of 20 shortly after the stroke but that there was a marked improvement on average 108 days after the stroke (eight patients scored below 17 and two patients scored 18, where <17 = pathological, 17-18 is a borderline score). One aspect is clear that ten out of ten patients were aprexic immediately following the stroke, there was marked improvement on average 108 days later, even though eight out of the ten patients' aprexie remained at a pathological level. Still it is not clear in this research exactly what therapeutic measures were taken in order to improve the aprexic score.

It can be concluded that Aprexia can be defined as the inability to make use of the normal tools of daily life or to imitate gesturesThis may result from a spatiotemporal destruction of learned movement or the inability visually to interpret an object or gesture. Hemiplegic subjects with aprexa will experience difficulty in using the tools of daily living such as a spoon, a fork or a tooth brush and they will have extra difficulty in learning new tool use or new tasks, like using a wheel chair or relearning basic functional tasks and caring for themselves. The most damaging effect of aprexa may be that subjects suffering from this condition will fail to obtain the appropriate stimulations necessary for neural recovery.

3. Memory dysfunction:

Re-learning motor functions following a stroke involves the storage and retrieval of information. As in the case of a defective memory, patients are unable to store and retrieve valuable information about the motor learning process, which can hamper their ability to acquire motor skills. According to Hochstenbach and Mulder (1999) patients with severe memory disorder in fact live in *vacuo* and are no longer able to profit from the available information. The memory function also has an essential role in the plastic reorganisation of the neurons within the damaged brain. The following discussion examines some of the consequences of memory impairment following a stroke.

It is therefore important to distinguish between memory and attention because both these conditions may interfere with the learning capacity of hemiplegic subjects. People with attention disorder have difficulty in registering, and processing information, whereas memory problems will interfere with the storage and retrieval of information. It should also be noted that in the process of storing different information, the attention function plays a crucial role. Attention processes guide the selective pick-up of information, and memory processes are responsible for the storage of this information (Hochstenbach and Mulder, 1999). Many patients whose learning abilities are impaired, claim to have a good 'memory'; because the early recollections seem so vivid and easy to retrieve (Lezak 1995). The author further suggests that other patients who complain of memory problems actually have disorders of attention or mental tracking that interfere with learning and recall but are in themselves distinguishable from those with memory function. It thus seems important to identify the exact nature of the disorder, and distinguish between attention and memory dysfunction that is hindering factor in the process of motor relearning.

Short-term memory plays a crucial role in decision making, problem solving, movement production and evaluation (Hochstenbach and Mulder 1999). Most damaging effect of short-term memory can be its interfering effect on motor relearning process; given that the therapy instructions may be lost before they can be implemented. In many stroke patients, whose short-term memory is affected, these problems are structural: messages are forgotten or a conversation cannot be followed, so that therapy instructions can be totally or partially lost even before they are to be used (Hochstenbach and Mulder 1999). Moreover the short-term memory along with attention plays a crucial role in transform experience into knowledge. Since storage in short-term memory is transient, so to use the information in the future it is necessary for the selected information to be transferred into a long-term memory store (Hochstenbach and Mulder 1999). It is clear that if information is already lost in the short-term memory it will never reach the long-term memory. Therefore people with short-term memory problems will experience difficulty in relearning different muscle function and reacquisition of functional autonomy. Yet in fact they can retrieve those functions already stored in the early stages of skill acquisition. This would suggest that hemiplegic subjects with an intact long-term memory may use functional exercises. Therefore it would be more appropriate to use functional exercise like standing up and getting in and out of the bed or walking as a means to relearn the motor functions. Unfortunately this retrieval process may itself be impaired, in which case the hemiplegic subject may no longer able to retrieve the memory of stored functional skills with the result that they fail to perform simple tasks like standing up and walking. These difficulties are not linked to motor or sensory impairment but rather due to the difficulty in retrieving the memory of different functional skills from storage.

A deficient memory can not only seriously impede the reacquisition of motor functions but it can also have an adverse effect on the process of neurogenesis. The function of memory plays an important role in the process of retention and maturation of newly proliferated neurons and thus an impaired memory in the wake of a stroke may hinder this process. Gould et al (1999) suggest that granule neurons produced in adulthood are necessary for hipocampal activity in certain types of learning and memory. It follows that an impaired memory both hinders the relearning of motor functions while at the same time itself contributing to an insufficient neural recovery.

Harris and Sunderland (1981) conducted a survey of the management of memory disorder in rehabilitation units in the United Kingdom. The result showed that out of the fifteen stroke patients fourteen needed help and advice on memory problems. One of the drawbacks of this research was that there were only 22 responses out of 49 questionnaires distributed. The result showed that respondents were using a wide range of tests, training procedures and aids. This research does not elucidate the interaction of impaired memory on motor relearning, nor does it explore the possible compensatory measures that were adapted by the respondents in the motor relearning process. However one aspect at least is clear from this study, namely that a large number of people suffer from memory dysfunction as a result of a stroke. According to Hochstenbach and Mulder (1999) (re) learning skills are totally dependent on memory, which is to say, on the capacity to retain information about ongoing actions and events. Therefore it is obvious that a rehabilitation strategy has to be adapted in the event of memory dysfunction. One important aspect to consider in this case is that memory has different aspects, such as short-term or long term memory, declarative memory or episodic memory. It can normally be assumed that all the aspects of memory may not be impaired and so patients with memory dysfunction may use the intact aspect of their memory function to compensate the aspect that is impaired. This may involve an evaluation and then the identification of the intact aspect of memory. The therapist can then use this intact component of the memory to obtain the therapeutic goal, instead of adopting a ready-made therapeutic technique. For example, Prigatano (1988) states that asking for actions related to memories with an emotional content will often lead to better results than asking for the performance of separate movements in *vacuo*.

In conclusion, the memory function is essential for the storage and retrieval of information and experience. Re-learning movements and functional tasks involves storing and retrieving this information and it is for this reason that hemiplegic subjects with memory dysfunction will experience difficulty in regaining their functional autonomy. Moreover memory function and learning play an important role in the retention and maturation of newly proliferated neurons and so neural recovery will be hindered in hemiplegic subjects with an impaired memory function.

Here it is important to distinguish between memory and attention – the memory function is involved in the process of storing and retrieving information, whereas the attention function is used in the process of processing and registering that information. Moreover there are different aspects of memory function, which include short-term and long term memory, declarative memory or episodic memory. It is therefore important to identify which aspect of the memory is impaired and then the rehabilitation strategy has to be adapted accordingly.

4. Disorder in the selection and evaluation of input (Hemi-neglect):

Hemi-neglect or unilateral neglect or hemi-inattention is one of the most prominent examples of a selection and representational deficit. These patients are often identified as patients with hemi-neglect or hemi inattention. In fact, they suffer from a disorder in the selection and evaluation of input received by the affected hemi corps. According to Hochstenbach and Mulder (1999) hemi-neglect is an attentional or representational deficit leading to the available information being ignored. Robertson et al (1993) defines unilateral neglect as a failure, difficulty, or slowness in reporting or interacting with objects (or sounds or representations) in the contra-lateral hemi-space (most frequently) left space, as right-hemisphere lesions are more common in people with hemi-neglect.

Hemiplegic subjects with right hemisphere damage often have hemi-neglect, depending on the area of the hemisphere that is affected. Robertson et al (1993) suggest that the neglect is due to an acquired damage to structures of the right hemisphere (usually) including the parietal lobe, dorso-lateral and medial frontal lobes, and the portion of reticular formation. In this context Vallar (1993) affirms that in unilateral neglect there is a range of brain areas that appear to be implicated, though the parietal lobe is particularly important. Moreover unilateral hemi-neglect is often further complicated due to the presence of hemi-anopsia (the absence of half of the visual field) and or due to the presence of an impaired deep and superficial sensation on the affected side. However hemi-neglect due to visual and sensory impairment does not fall in the category of cognitive impairment and according to Diller and Weinberg (1977); De Renzi (1978) Halligan et al (1997) the presence of homonymous hemi-anopia seems to increase the likelihood of visual neglect. Bisiach and Vallar (1988) suggest that hemi-neglect cannot be explained by a deficit of sensory or motor functions, but rather involves a range of phenomena related to the high-level representation of space and spatial perception.

Rizzolatti et al (1987) have explained that multiple and dissociable spatial frames of reference exist in both animals and humans. These include personal space, near personal area within reach and extra personal area at a distance and all these areas can be either collectively or individually impaired. It is therefore clear that hemi-neglect or hemi-inattention is a complex disorder of attention and perception of one side of the body, which may be further complicated due to the presence of somato-sensory, motor and visual defects.

Complex bi-directional relationships exist between perception and attention (Robertson et al 1993). They further suggest that these perception and attention systems may be responsible for generating bilateral and alternative signals of activation and inhibition during different functional activities. That is, when one side of the body is excited, the brain sends an inhibitory impulse to the other side of the body and vice versa. An imbalance of this bidirectional function of the brain can complicate hemi-neglect, which in turn may produce abnormal motor activities, like the pushing syndrome.

During a normal functional act like walking or getting in and out of the bed when one side of the body is activated, simultaneously there may be inhibition on the other side of the body. Now in a damaged brain this inhibiting effect on the unaffected side is absent. The cause of persistent neglect is due to an inhibition of the attentional networks in the damaged hemisphere by the intact hemisphere (Robertson et al 1993). Consequently, instead of a bilateral and alternate activation and inhibition, there might be a simple activation and activation on the unaffected side; at the same time inhibition and inhibition on the affected side of the body, which result hyperactivity on the unaffected side or a pushing syndrome. The impairment of this bilateral mechanism of alternate activation and inhibition can cause the pushing syndrome; which is when subjects with hemi-neglect try to perform functional tasks with their affected side and there is an exaggerated activity of the unaffected side causing a further inhibition of the affected side. It seems that a combination of disorders of perception and attention in the hemi-corps may result in hemi-inattention and this can prove to be the principal barrier to attaining functional autonomy for many hemiplegic subjects.

Robertson and North (1994) compared the effect of bilateral limb movements with those of unilateral ones on the left side and discovered that an improvement in neglect produced by unilateral movements was eliminated when both hands were moved together. Here it is suggested that the underlying reason for this is that activation of the limb operates by means of a process of alternate inhibition and excitation, in which case bilateral limb movements may help to reduce hemi-neglect or hemi-inattention. However it is not clear how much of this improvement can be attributed to spontaneous recovery and how much should be attributed to appropriately planned exercise. In practice a large majority of stroke patients display an absence of movement on the affected side, which may render it difficult to perform bilateral alternative movements. Still in many hemiplegic subjects, it may possible to use bilateral movement of different segments, such as bilateral movements of the scapula, the shoulder, the hip or the knee.

It can thus be concluded that hemi-neglect or hemi-inattention is a disorder in the selection and representation deficit of input received by the affected hemi-corps. It is also a failure, difficulty or slowness in reporting or interacting with objects. This may be due to damage of the complex bi-directional relationship that exists in the brain between perception and action. This bi-directional relation is responsible for the bilateral and alternate activation and inhibition of movement during the execution of different functional tasks. The cause of this persistent neglect is an inhibition by the intact hemisphere of the attention networks in the damaged hemisphere (Robertson et al 1993).

5. Attention disorder:

Attention forms an important part of the cognitive system. Zomeren and Brower (1994) define attention as a cognitive state characterised by a selective bias for processing certain internal and external stimuli. They further suggest that the important aspects of attention in this respect are selectivity, intensity, and its dynamic character. According to Theeuwis (1992) attention is essential to the correct perception of conjunctions, though unattended features are often conjoined prior to their conscious perception. This top down feature is capable of utilizing past experience and contextual information. The attention system has an important role to perform in registering and processing all information received. An impaired capacity of attention can have serious consequences on neural recovery and attaining functional autonomy. The following discussion examines briefly the different aspects of attention, looking at the part of the brain responsible for the attention function, as well as its importance for neural recovery and reacquisition of motricity.

Van Zomeren and Brouwer (1994) describe the attention system as having four distinct parts, comprising selective, focused, divided and sustained attention. These distinctive features of the system of attention are explained as follows:

- Selective attention reflects our capacity to distinguish one source of stimulus from another.
- Focused attention enables us to direct the attention to the main aspect of a task without being distracted by irrelevant stimuli.
- Divided attention reflects our capacity to shift between several input sources or tasks and to do two or more things simultaneously.
- Sustained attention reflects the ability to concentrate on a given task over long and generally unbroken periods of time without a substantial decline or large fluctuation in the performance.

Van Zomeren and Brouwer (1994) suggest that these aspects of the mechanism of attention may experience significant disruption as the result of a stroke, leading to a decline in flexibility, together with difficulties in concentrating on a task for a prolonged period. They further note that a fundamental aspect of attention concerns the speed of information processing and almost all stroke patients demonstrate a substantial decline in this respect, which results in a general slowing of thinking as well as of acting. It is therefore essential first to identify the attention subsystem that remains intact and then to use this part of the system as the basis for rehabilitation. It is clear that many people after a stroke have impaired attention function, and which can severely disrupt the relearning of motor function and reacquisition of functional autonomy.

Van Zomeren and Brouwer (1994) describe how the cerebral cortex has three different functions in attention, activation, localisation, and analysis. These three roles are respectively as follows:

- The cerebral cortex itself serves as a source of input for the brainstem reticular formation as a regulator of activation.
- The cortex functions as the final destination of signals that are otherwise not attended to.
- The cortex further supplies a representation of the outside world to localise new and arousing stimuli.

Mesulam (1985) describes that the frontal lobes may be particularly important in the regulation of what he calls the overall attentional tone. Moreover the cerebral cortex functions as the analyser or, better, the repository of sensory input. Heilman and Van den Abell (1979) concluded from their study that the right hemisphere appears to dominate the activation of attention and thus it is not difficult to understand that hemiplegic subjects with right hemisphere damage often experience a form of attention disorder.

Furthermore, the basal ganglia and limbic system, in particularly the afferent part of basal ganglia, which consists of the caudate nucleus and putamen, are probably involved in the selective component of attention. Luria (1973) describes that the hippocampus and the caudate nucleus are the essential structures for the elimination of responses to irrelevant stimuli, enabling an organism to behave in a strictly selective manner, and thus a lesion in these structures is a source of the breakdown of behavioural selectivity. This impaired selectivity may result in slowness in the processing of information. Hochtenbach and Mulder (1999) note that almost all stroke patients reveal a substantial decrease in the speed of information processing, resulting in a general slowing of thought and action. Patients often notice a loss of automaticity and fluency with the result that they have to control every act consciously (Fasotti and Kovacs 1995).

The function of attention not only serves to regulate behavioural selectivity, but it is also responsible for the selectivity of the motor function. This can be seen as a perceptual filtering out of all but one single input source on the basis of task and context variables, as well as the physical characteristics of the input sources(s) (Hochtenbach and Mulder 1999). For example the act of getting out of a chair consists of the flexion of the trunk and lower limbs, followed by an extension of the limbs and trunk, all of which involves multiple and complex movements. Attention and perception enables one to perform this complex task relatively smoothly by activating one group while inhibiting the others, by prioritising and filtering muscle action and eventually this complex action of the muscles is transformed into a simple functional task. It follows that an impaired system of attention can be responsible for slowness in performing such functional tasks, which in extreme cases can even extend to the impossibility of executing the task in hand. Therefore the functional impairment in hemiplegic subjects does not only result from impaired motor and sensory function but it also result from impaired attention function.

The capacity to learn different motor skills may be severely reduced in stroke patients with attention disorder. Hochtenbach and Mulder (1999) state that attention forms not only a prerequisite for almost all human action and is thus of crucial importance for effective human behaviour and survival, but it also plays a major role in the (re) acquisition of skills. Memory is involved in retention of information or experience, which it then retrieves as needed, whereas the attention system is involved in the process of retaining different information or experience. With an impaired attention function this information and experience will not be processed and will thus be lost without being retained in the long term memory. As it was mentioned earlier this process of attention guides the selective pick-up of information, and memory processes are responsible for the storage of this information (Hochstenbach and Mulder 1999). In other words, in the course of transforming short term memory into long term memory the function of attention plays a crucial role. Hemiplegic subjects with an impaired attention function will thus be unable to learn and integrate different therapeutic activities to readapt with the functional loss. Again the disability will depend on the severity of attention dysfunction and the presence of other cognitive and sensoriomotor problem.

Experience-dependent change within the damaged neural circuits is largely dependent on the intact attention function. Robertson et al (1997) suggest that the attention systems of the brain have a privileged role in recovery following brain damage. According to Recanzone et al (1993) experience-dependent plastic reorganisation depends on attention being paid by the recipient to the stimulation responsible for such changes. It can be assumed that a failure to facilitate experience-dependent change, which results from impaired attention function, may hinder the process of neural recovery. Different experiences received during therapeutic activities may not be able to produce change in the intact neural circuits in hemiplegic subjects with impaired attention function; consequently there would be no change in their functional status as well. In other words, hemiplegic subjects with impaired attention will be unable to process and register information and so it can be extremely difficult for them to relearn motor function and to regain functional autonomy. However the attention system has different aspects; like selective attention, focused attention, divided attention and sustained attention; 'which attention systems are necessary for experience-dependent reorganisation and how it is that they are necessary component for such reorganisation is not clear' (Robertson 1999). More research is also necessary to understand better the nature and interactions among the independent and supramodal attentional systems of the brain.

It can thus be concluded that the attention function plays an important role in processing and integrating different experience and information and then transform them into knowledge. In other words attention function is crucial to transforming short-term memory into the long-term memory store. Subjects with attention dysfunction may not be able to integrate these different motor learning activities. Moreover attention has a privileged role in facilitating experience-dependent functional reorganisation in the intact neural circuits of a damaged brain. It follows that any impairment of the attention function in hemiplegic subjects may severely affect their ability to relearn motor functions and regain functional autonomy.

Summary of cognitive dysfunction in people following stroke:

Impaired cognitive dysfunction can severely affect hemiplegic subjects in the process of relearning of motor function and regaining functional autonomy. The repercussions of different cognitive dysfunctions can include:
- Cognitive function have important role in relearning of motor function.
- Relevance information and then rehearsing them constitute important ingredient for transforming information into knowledge.
- Attention and memory are two important cognitive functions, which are essential for this transforming process; irrelevant information can remain unattended and may not reach into memory to be stored as knowledge.
- In case of impaired attention the available information will remain unattended, and they will neither reach short-term nor long-term memory; therefore the unateended information cannot be transformed into knowledge.
- Functional activities constitute relevant information for the brain individual muscle activities do not.
- Some cognitive dysfunctions hinder the process of neural recovery.
- And finally executive function plays a crucial role in leading an independent and purposeful life.

Five common cognitive dysfunctions in hemiplegic subjects and their repercussions:

1. Executive function:
- The executive function is important for planning, taking initiative and the performance of purposeful activities.
- Depending on the severity of executive dysfunction and the presence of other cognitive dysfunctions, hemiplegics can be dependent on other people for various activities of daily life.

- Despite the recovery of muscle function and the reacquisition of functional autonomy, the hemiplegic subjects with impaired executive function may remain dependent on other people for the activities of daily living.
- The passive living condition in people with executive dysfunction may severely hinder the possibility of neural recovery.

2. Apraxia:
- Apraxia is the inability to use the tools of daily life or to imitate gestures.
- This may result from the loss of the ability to situate learned movement in a spatiotemporal framework or to provide visual interpretation of an object or gesture.
- Hemiplegic subjects with apraxa will experience difficulty in using the tools of daily life, such as a spoon, a fork or a tooth brush, and they will have extra difficulty in learning to use new tools, like a wheel chair.
- The most damaging effect of apraxa may be the failure to provide appropriate stimulations necessary for neural recovery.

3. Memory:
- Memory involves the storage and retrieval of information and experience.
- Hemiplegic subjects with memory dysfunction will experience difficulty to relearn motor functions and to regain functional autonomy.
- Memory function and learning play an important role in bringing to maturity and the retention of newly produced neurons and thus neural recovery will be hindered in hemiplegic subjects with an impaired memory function.
- It is important to distinguish between memory and attention – the memory function is involved in the process of storing and retrieving information, whereas the attention function finds its place in the processing and registering of information.

- The different aspects of memory function, which includes short-term, long-term, declarative and procedural memory, and it is important identifying which aspect of the memory is impaired and which is intact in planning a rehabilitation strategy.

4. Selection and representational deficit or hemi-neglect:
    - Hemi-neglect or hemi-inattention is the disorder affecting the selection and treatment of input received by the hemi corps.
    - It is also reflected in any failure, difficulty or slowness in reporting or interacting with objects.
    - This may be due to damage of the complex bi-directional relationship within the brain that exists between perception and attention.
    - This bidirectional relation is responsible for the bilateral and alternate activation and inhibition of the motor function.
    - The cause of persistent neglect is an inhibition by the intact hemisphere of the networks controlling attention in the damaged hemisphere (Robertson et al 1993).

5. Attention:
    - Attention is a cognitive state characterised by a selective bias for processing certain internal and external stimuli.
    - This consists of four different aspects, those of selective, focused, divided and sustained attention.
    - Defective selectivity in the motor function resulting from an impaired attention function can cause slowness in task performance, which in severe cases can render it difficult or in severe case impossibility to perform functional task.
    - Attention function plays an important role in the processing and integration experience and information within the knowledge base and so an impaired attention function can hinder relearning of muscle function and regaining of functional autonomy in hemiplegic subjects.

> - Experience-dependent functional reorganisation in the brain is dependent on the attention function and thus an impaired capacity of attention will disrupt neuro- remodelling activities following a stroke.

Some strategies to minimise the interfering effects of different cognitive dysfunctions in hemiplegic subjects:

Cognitive dysfunction in people after a stroke can hinder the process of relearning of muscle function and regaining of functional anatomy. The severity of the hindering effect is dependent on the extent of cognitive dysfunction. The most devastating effect of cognitive dysfunction is that it can impede the neural remodelling process. The brain is deprived of necessary stimulation required to facilitate neural recovery in people with cognitive dysfunction. In other words hemiplegic subjects with impaired cognitive function can be considered as living in a stimulation deprived environment. It is therefore important to identify possible strategies to minimise the interfering effects of cognitive dysfunction. The following discussion examines some possible strategies to minimise the effects of executive dysfunction, aprexia, memory dysfunction, hemi-neglect, and attention disorder on relearning motor skills and attaining functional autonomy.

<u>Possible strategies to cope with executive dysfunction</u>: People with executive dysfunction are dependent on others for many of the activities of daily life. Here they often experience difficulty with both planning and execution. It would seem that one appropriate strategy would therefore consist in the performance of these functional activities in a routine manner, which is to say undertaking the same function at the same time every day. It has often been observed that elderly people are obsessively ritualistic in their daily routine and this might simply be a natural strategy to cope with the age related impairment of the executive function. This ritualism in activities of daily life develops progressively as the executive function deteriorates. In hemipligic subjects with an impaired executive function, the same strategy can be adapted to help them to cope with the resultant difficulties of daily life. Repeating these tasks, that is, performing

the same task in the same manner may serve to foster a functional reorganisation in the intact neural circuits of the damaged brain and eventually this would help the patient to cope with dysexecutive syndrome. In contrast, if they become dependent on others for the performance of these tasks then the intact neural circuits risk being deprived of the experience needed for change.

Lezak (1982) explains that there are four steps in goal-directed behaviour: - one has to formulate a goal or an intention; - one has to plan the different steps needed to achieve the goal; —one has to translate this plan into purposeful action, which requires the ability to initiate, maintain, adjust and stop the ongoing activity; and —one has to perform effectively. It is important to evaluate which aspect of this goal directed behaviour is impaired, and which aspect is still intact, and then to organise a plan to overcome the difficulties linked to this impaired executive function. That is to say, if the patient has only a problem with the formulation of goals, then it may be appropriate to define these goals for them, thus allowing them to take steps and translate the plan into purposive action. Whereas if they are able to formulate the goal but have problems with planning and then translating this plan into purposive action, then it might be helpful to design a cognitive map (a visual representation) of the different steps needed to achieve the goals of everyday living. However, in the absence of convincing evidence, the effectiveness of this type of strategy to attain functional autonomy remains unproven. Moreover, the problem of hemiplegic subjects may be further complicated due the presence of other associated cognitive and sensorio-motor deficiencies.

It can be supposed that hemiplegic subjects with executive functional disorder will tend to perform the tasks of daily living in a stereotyped manner, which is to say executing the same task in the same way every day. There are in fact four steps to goal-directed behaviour: (1) formulating the goal, (2) planning the different steps needed, (3) translating this plan into action, and finally (4) performing them effectively. It follows that identifying which aspect of the goal directed behaviour is impaired and which intact is a necessary prerequisite to developing a strategy to overcome this dysexecutive syndrome.

Overcoming the difficulties linked with apraxia: Apraxa is impairment in the reproduction of learned gestures, which is reflected in a difficulty in imitating movements, in executing isolated movements of the limb, and in using the tools necessary in daily living. Ietswaart et al (2001) affirm that this disorder cannot be explained as a deficit of elementary movement or intellectual deterioration or poor language comprehension. They further state that in the case of apraxia stored perceptual information may be unavailable to the frontal systems, which are responsible for producing movement. Here the subjects do not know how to perform certain functions or to use certain objects. For example, they no longer know what to do with a toothbrush or how to use a knife and fork. Moreover, Hu et al (1999) suggest that in apraxia there may be reduced accuracy where reaching an object with the ipsilateral hand in the absence of visual feedback. Still any difficulty in reaching an object without visual feedback may also be due to impairment in either the profound or the superficial sensation. It follows that the sensory problems of the patient need to be evaluated before diagnosing apraxia. Therefore Ietswaart et al (2001) suggest that apraxia should preclude any substantive motor deficit as the cause for failure in a task of gesture reproduction. Milner and Goodale (1995) also state that some apraxic symptoms, such as the impaired imitation of gesture, could be interpreted in terms of disconnection between the dorsal and visual pathways. Aprexia is a cognitive deficit where the learned gestures and experiences of tool use are no longer available to the frontal system of the brain, resulting in difficulty to use different tools of daily living and imitate a gesture. These difficulties exclude any difficulty that results from sensory, motor, other cognitive or language comprehension difficulty.

Since the motor system is disconnected from the representation and appearance of specific actions and their related sense, so it cannot access the sensoriomotor control and its associated motor cortices of the frontal lobes, which will in turn serve to aggravate the symptoms of apraxia. Where this condition itself is responsible for the impaired motor function and the incapacity to perform functional activities, it is reasonable to recreate the perceptual information of tool use and perform gesture using the exiting intact sensory and motor function.

However in the presence of motor and sensory impairment, the minimising of aprexia may be difficult.

It can be concluded that people with apprexia will be unable to use many of the tools of daily living or to imitate gestures, which may be due to the destruction of the perceptual interpretation of the knowledge acquired in the utilisation of the object or the production of movement. This impairment may be aggravated due to the presence of motor, sensory and other cognitive dysfunctions. Here one strategy might be to recreate a new perceptual interpretation of the objects and tasks, using the still intact sensory and motor functions.

Some possible strategies to minimise the difficulty relearn motor function and regain functional autonomy in hemimlegic subjects with memory dysfunction:

Although hemiplegic subjects with impaired short-term memory can experience learning problems, they may still be able to improve different motor functions through the use of functional exercises like standing up, reaching for an object and walking around, etc. Given that these skills are acquired in the early stages of life, when the hemiplegic subjects will be aware of having performed them, no new learning process will be involved. According to Hochstenbach and Mulder (1999) it is procedural memory that deals with knowledge on how to perform activities, while declarative memory is responsible for factual knowledge. Selecting the most appropriate form of motor action involves the procedural memory system, whereas the performance of the action itself depends on the declarative memory (Hochstenbach and Mulder 1999). In the home environment where the subject is used to performing these tasks, the procedural memory is more vivid as compared with a novel environment, such as a physiotherapy department or in a hospital. It is thus more suitable to organise the re-education of hemiplegic subjects with memory dysfunction at home, where they can practice different tasks like walking, standing up and getting in and out of bed. It can be assumed that the repetition of such functional movements may result in a reorganisation of the intact neural circuits, where the procedural memory can progressively play a more dominant role in the re-learning process. However, the acquisition of new skills, like learning to use a wheel chair, can involve using both short-term and long-term memory, as well as the function of attention. It should also be noted that if the patients have a deficient declarative memory, they might not be able to transform their learned action into purposeful activities of daily living. Tulving (1972) has made the distinction between episodic and semantic memory, where the former refers to the memory of personal experience and its temporal context, whereas semantic memory is the system for receiving, retaining, and transmitting information about the meaning of words and classification of concepts. It is thus important to discover which aspect of the memory is impaired and then use the intact part of the memory to compensate this memory loss. During muscle re-education in hemiplegic subjects with impaired short-term memory, it is important to use functional movement, as for example standing up, reaching for an object, transfer training and early walking practice etc, and those tasks would be learnt more effectively within home in people with intact procedural memory. However, there is paucity of research-based evidence to support the efficacy of this type of measure as a means of overcoming memory impairment.

Emotional information is better than neutral content, since it serves to raise the level of conscious awareness and this aspect of memory can also be used in therapy (Hochstenbach and Mulder 1999). Prigatano (1988) described a number of examples in which the recollection of past feelings in brain-damaged patients led to a more realistic self-perception and powerfully reinforced the experience. Both memory and learning are context-dependent, meaning that an important factor in the retention of motor skills is the relationship between the context of practice and the context of application. Tulving and Thomson (1973) showed that more the context of the final application resembles the context of practice, the better the retention performance will be. Hence, it is important to realise that the recollection of movement contained in memory provides not only motor related information, but also all the contextual information associated with the movement (Hochstenbach and Mulder 1999).

Hemiplegic subjects with memory dysfunction are unable to store and retrieve information as needed, which may severely hinder their learning capabilities. However people with intact procedural memory may still preserve an intact recollection of various functional tasks stored during the early stage of skill acquisition. It thus seems evident that using functional activities may be an appropriate strategy to relearn motor function. In contrast learning new tasks like the use of a wheel chair or performing individual muscle functions may prove extremely difficult for those with an impaired short-term memory.

<u>Possible coping strategy for hemi-inattention:</u> One strategy may be to move objects around in the room as a way to overcome the problem linked to hemi-neglect. This involves placing the object in question on the neglected side so that the patient has to turn towards this side during the performance of different activities. Studies carried out by Azouvie (1997a); Azouvie (1997b) and Robertson et al (1993) have had favourable results where the objects were placed on the affected side, though on condition that the patients receive at least twenty hours therapy. These studies all used a similar type of therapy by placing objects on the neglected side in order to provide the maximum stimulation on the affected side. However, it must be said that two other studies (Bergego et al 1997 and Robertson et al 1990), which used a similar type of activity, produced negative results, though here the duration of therapy in both cases was relatively short. Visual stimulation on the neglected side may indeed improve the field of vision, but seems more appropriate for the problems related to lateral hemi-anopia. Meanwhile Bergego et al (1997) and Robertson et al (1990) have observed that the awareness of the neglected part of the body is improved in subjects, whose lateral visual neglect is reduced. The subject's ability to supply visual information to the motor system may help to improve the awareness of the neglected part of the body. This may explain the underlying reason for the positive results contained in the above studies. It is important to remember that the hemi-neglect is a cognitive impairment, which reduces attention and perception of one side of the body.

According to Bisiach and Vallar (1988) this form of neglect can occur separately on the left side of the body, without affecting awareness of external space on the left side, and vice versa. The pre-motor theory of attention proposed by Rizzolati and Camarada

(1987) suggests that the process of attention is only possible due to the activation of the neural circuits involved in motor preparation. Thus, attention works to enhance the importance of that which is intended as a target for action. Visual control of the target will facilitate the attention and thus activate the neural circuits responsible for motor preparation. Moreover, visual control helps to eliminate irrelevant inputs that can have an inhibiting effect on the activation of the neural circuits. Undertaking movement without visual control may help to reduce visio-spatial neglect, especially when the patient performs the movement in the neglected space. Ladavas et al (1997) suggest that conducting even small movements with the left hand on the left side of space produces a significant reduction in visio-spatial neglect and this applies even when the hands are out of sight. Therefore it is important to perform exercises on the affected limb without visual control, which may help to minimise subjects of both visual and corporal neglect.

Often the symptoms of hemi-neglect can experience an abrupt remission following another stroke on the opposite hemisphere. Sprague (1966) found that a strong spatial bias in cats caused by a large unilateral posterior lesion could be improved by destroying the superior colliculus on the side opposite to the initial visual input. Even though the more florid manifestations usually remit in the large majority of patients who show acute signs of the disorder following a stroke in the right hemisphere, according to Klara et al (1997), this is a condition that actually has long-lasting and severe effects in other areas, such as the recovery of motor function. There are several explanations of this partial or complete reduction of hemi-neglect following a second stroke. Whatever the cause of this remission of symptoms, it is clear that there exists a latent functional capacity in the damaged hemisphere which needs to be explored. Robertson (1993) suggests that in the case of hemi-neglect latent functions exist in the damaged hemisphere that can only be unlocked with an alteration to the dynamic architecture of the brain's systems of attention and orientation. He further insists on the importance of analysing the cognitive architecture of spatial attention and has suggested two types of rehabilitative processes: the joint activation of mutually facilitating networks, and the reduction of inhibitory competition. As already noted, movements of the left hand in the left space can significantly reduce left visuo-spatial neglect as well. Most probably the movements of the left arm on the left hemi-space activate the neural circuit on the right hemisphere (lesioned hemisphere), while at the same time inhibiting the competitor neural circuits of the left hemisphere. Robertson (1999) affirms that by inducing the subject to make voluntary movements with the left hand in the left hemispace, it is possible that the left half of the somato-sensory spatial sector is activated. It has been observed that patients with left hemi-neglect are unable to maintain the standing position, but this is considerably improved if they perform left handed movements in the left space while in this position. Similarly, it has been shown that when patients with hemi-neglect perform bilateral hand movements (alternative opening and clenching the fists for example) during walking, this can improve their ability to walk. This is most probably because the movements of the hand in the neglected hemi-space activate the facilitating network, while at the same time reducing the activation of inhibitory competition, which in turn serves to improve the patient's capacity to maintain standing position or walk. Still there is no research-based evidence to validate this hypothesis. Moreover, this also goes against the conventional physiotherapy practice in which patients cross their fingers in bringing the arm towards the midline of the body, while performing different activities like standing up and walking etc. According to Robertson (1999) some non-science based orthodoxies in rehabilitation maintain that motor rehabilitation should always be conducted bilaterally, that is with the 'good' arm always 'helping' the hemi-paretic limb. He further affirms that whatever the virtues of this approach with non-neglect patients, it is clear that such a blanket recommendation for the neglect patients would be misleading. At least some of the time, the lesioned hemisphere must be given the opportunity to activate the disabling competition from the other half of the brain. Moreover, when patients with spasticity, whose voluntary movements are dominated by involuntary muscular contraction and exaggerated reflex activity, it is important for them to practice holding their spastic arm with the unaffected hand in an inhibited position in order to prevent the strengthening of the spastic pattern.

It can be concluded that it is important to provide visual stimulation by placing different objects on the affected side and subjects with hemi-neglect must learn to be aware of the neglected part during the different activities of daily living. Furthermore, during different therapy like standing up and re-education for walking, patients should be encourage to perform movements of the neglected limb, like bilateral and alternative opening and closing of the fists while for example trying to stand up or while walking.

By way of conclusion, it may be said that in the case of hemi-inattention it is useful to make adjustments in the room, such as placing objects on the neglected side, which helps to reduce visual neglect and eventually improves the awareness of the neglected part of the body. Performing movements in the neglected space can also help to minimise corporal neglect. This attention function plays an important role in the generation of bilateral and alternating movements, and hemi-neglect is a combination of attention and perception dysfunction. It follows that encouraging bilateral alternative movements may serve to minimise lateral hemi-inattention.

IX

Strategies to Minimise the Difficulty to Relearning Muscle Function in People with Attention Dysfunction

One of the important roles of attention is to facilitate an experience-dependent change in the intact neural circuit of brain cells. Kempermann et al (1988) describe how animals kept in an enriched as compared to an impoverished environment show cell genesis in the hippocampus. Moreover, as has already been mentioned, the undertaking a program of planned experience for hemiplegic patients can facilitate experience-dependent changes in the intact neural circuits of the brain, while enhancing the survival of newly generated brain cells,. However, patients with attention disorder may be unable to benefit from the experience received and the program would thus fail to facilitate any change in the intact neural circuit. The therapeutic activities will not exert any impact on patients if they are unable to pay attention to the stimulation received. Robartson (1999) suggests that rehabilitation of attention function is important as an intervening step in rehabilitating other type of cognitive, motor, and perceptual function, given that attention is a key element in of experience-dependent plastic reorganisation. There are several aspects of attention function; according to Van Zomeren and Brouwer (1994) these include 'selective attention, focused attention, divided attention and sustained attention'. According to Robertson (1999) the question of whether and how the selective attention, attentional switching can be rehabilitated is still open.

It seems important to find which aspect of attention is impaired and then utilise the intact attention sub-system in order to obtain the desired therapeutic goal to improve muscle function. Van Zomeren and Brower (1994) further suggest that the main point of this stimulation is to alleviate attention impairment through the direct stimulation of the brain structures involved in any particular aspect attention. Treatment is based on submitting patients to repetitive exercises and providing them with feedback about their performance. For example in people whose selective attention is impaired who cannot prioritise muscle function in a selective basis during a functional task may use focus attention and learn to pay attention toward the impaired aspect of the muscle function to minimise difficulty. It may be appropriate hemiplegic people with impaired selective attention, to stress on individual muscle exercise with maximum attention is given towards individual muscle function before progress to perform functional exercise, while maintaining focus on the task performance. In contrast a hemiplegic subject with intact selective attention may use functional exercise to improve task performance, unless certain individual muscle cannot participate during functional exercise, in which case more stress is given to improve those individual muscles until they can participate during functional task. In practice hemiplegic subjects should practice simple tasks like standing up and moving from the bed to a chair, or even if possible walking. That is to say, the task itself has to be simple so that the subject can concentrate on one task at a time. The subject must pay maximum attention to the task in hand and repeats them until this 'mental muscle' is properly developed and the experience of the task is transformed into knowledge of task performance. Sometimes isolation is important when relearning tasks in subjects with attention dysfunction and in this case the experience of working in a group or in a crowded physiotherapy department can have destructive effect on function of attention.

Whatever strategy is adapted whether it is individual muscle exercise in case of impaired selective attention or functional exercise with intact selective attention it is important that the exercise are active and repetitive. Repeated stimulation of the brain structure would normally facilitate neural growth or regeneration (Powell 1981) and attention would respond like a "mental muscle" whose function, as in the case of real muscles, could be improved by repeated exercise (Harris and Sunderland, 1981).

In conclusion the relearning of muscle function and regaining of functional autonomy can often be severely hindered in hemiplegic subjects with attention disorder. The attention function plays an important role in transferring experience into knowledge. Moreover experience-dependent plastic reorganisation depends on the attention being paid by the recipient to the stimulation responsible for such changes (Reconzone 1993). This attention function has four different aspects, which are (1) selective attention, (2) focused attention, (3) divided attention and (4) sustained attention. It is therefore important to identify which aspects of attention have been impaired and which remain intact. The use of a simple task, performed repeatedly and where the subject pays maximum attention on the task during this time, can be appropriate way to minimise the difficulties associated with attention impairment.

Conclusion: The importance of cognitive dysfunction and some alleviating measures have been discussed. However in reality cognitive dysfunction is not manifested in such a distinct way and hemiplegic subjects often present complex cognitive and sensorio-motor dysfunction. It is essential to understand the repercussion of each form of cognitive dysfunction on relearning motricity and attaining functional autonomy. Moreover it has been noted that certain forms of cognitive dysfunction are more dominant than others and thus cause a higher degree of interference. The repercussions of cognitive dysfunction must therefore be identified and the rehabilitation strategy adapted accordingly. It is also important to proceed with one form of cognitive dysfunction at a time, starting with predominant manifestation. Here it should be emphasised that if the stress of rehabilitation is only placed on muscular reinforcement or inhibiting spasticity through walking practice, without taking into account the barrier of cognitive dysfunction, then it can prove to be very difficult for both the patient and therapist alike.

Summary of strategies to minimise motor learning difficulties in people with different cognitive dysfunction following a stroke:

1. Executive dysfunction:
    - Hemiplegic subjects with impaired executive function may be able to learn to perform the tasks of daily life in a stereotypical manner, which is to say by performing the same task in the same way every day.
    - Hemiplegic subject with severely impaired executive function and in the presence of other cognitive dysfunction may be dependent on other people for the activities of daily living
    - There are four stages executive function or to achieve a goal-directed behaviour: (1) formulation of the goal, (2) planning the different step needed, (3) translate this plan into action, and finally (4) performing them effectively. Thus it seems important to start by identifying which aspect of the goal directed behaviour is impaired and which aspect is intact, and then conceiving a strategy to overcome the dysexecutive syndrome itself.
2. Apraxia:
    - Stroke victims with apraxia will be unable to use tools of everyday life or imitate gestures, which may be due to the loss of the perceptual interpretation of the techniques acquired in using the object or else to the inability to produce the movements required for its utilisation.
    - Here one strategy might be to recreate a new perceptual interpretation of the objects and the tasks performed with these objects, using the intact sensory and motor functions.
3. Memory dysfunction:
    - Hemiplegic subjects with memory dysfunction will be unable to store information and retrieve when needed, which can severely hinder the capacity to relearn motor function and regain functional autonomy.

- People with impaired short-term memory and with intact long-term memory may still preserve the memory of different functional tasks as those tasks were stored in the memory bank, in the early stage of skill acquisition. Therefore using functional tasks may be an appropriate strategy of reduction.
- However people with both short-term and long-term memory problems will experience extra difficulty in relearning the different motor functions.

4. Hemi-neglect:
    - It is useful to make adjustments in the room, such as placing objects on the neglected side, which helps to reduce visual neglect and eventually helps hemiplegic subjects to improve the awareness of the neglected part of the body.
    - Performing movement in the neglected space may also help to minimise corporal neglect.
    - Attention function plays an important role in generating bilateral and alternating movements. Hemi-neglect is the combination of attention and perception dysfunction and thus encouraging bilateral movement can help to minimise lateral hemi-neglect or hemi-inattention.

5. Attention dysfunction:
    - The function of attention plays an important role in transferring experience into knowledge and it is for this reason that relearning muscle function can be severely limited in people with attention dysfunction.
    - Experience-dependent plastic reorganisation depends on the attention being paid by the recipient to the stimulation responsible for such changes (Reconzone 1993) and so neural recovery can be restricted in people suffering from attention dysfunction.
    - Attention has four different aspects, which are (1) selective attention, (2) focused attention, (3) divided attention and (4) sustained attention. It is therefore important to identify which are the impaired and the intact aspects of attention.

> - The use of a simple task, performed repeatedly, while the subject is paying maximum attention can prove a useful strategy for minimising the difficulty of attention impairment.
> - Moreover individual muscle exercise may be more appropriate in people with impaired selective attention dysfunction; whereas functional exercises seems effective in people with intact selective attention, provided the individual muscles can participate during those functional tasks.

Secondary dysfunction of different contractile and non-contractile tissues and possible strategies to minimise these dysfunctions:

Impaired muscle function along with inactivity is not only responsible for structural change of the muscles but can also lead to widespread structural and functional change of different non-contractile tissues. As was stated in the chapter on the feedback control activities, muscle impairment following a stroke arises from two sources: one is the result of lesion itself and other is the result of secondary changes in the muscles themselves. Recent findings indicate that the most significant in terms of the effect on motor performance and functional activity are muscle weakness and the loss of motor control and these adaptive changes to the muscles and other soft tissues are major factors impacting negatively on recovery (Carr and Shepherd 2004). In mild cases there may be instability and pain in the joints, which in severe cases may lead to atrophy and contracture of the soft tissues along with joint deformity. In addition, changes in the structure and function of different tissues may eventually alter posture and balance reaction in hemiplegic subjects and can have a hindering effect on the recovery of functional autonomy. It is therefore essential to minimise structural and functional change in these muscles, as well as other non-contractile tissue. The following discussion will examine some of the consequences of inactivity on the structure and function of muscles, bone, ligament and cartilage before discussing possible measures to minimise these adverse effects.

Changes in muscle:

<u>The effects of inactivity on muscles:</u> Muscular inactivity due to the muscle paralysis may be responsible for muscle atrophy and weakness. A reduced level of activity leads to a stress deprivation of the muscles, which may be responsible for atrophy and degeneration of the different muscles. The following discussion reviews the underlying factors responsible for muscle atrophy in hemiplegic subjects.

According to Carr and Shepherd (2004) muscle weakness and fatigue will normally appear as a secondary consequence of disuse, when a person spends much of the day sitting and laying down. In a sedentary position these secondary changes are particularly evident in postural muscles, designed to counteract gravity since their natural role is no longer practised in this context. Stack et al (2006) state that an impairment of body structure and function is associated with the absence of exercises, such as walking about the home and community, moving from a lying to sitting or standing position, and turning around (Stack et al 2006). Atrophy of the quadriceps can appear as early as 3 days after immobilisation in normal individuals (Lindboe and Platou 1984). Halkjae-Kristensen and Ingeman-Hansen (1985) affirm that a 30% reduction of the cross-section area of quadriceps muscle fibres occurs within one month of immobilisation. This muscular atrophy may be accompanied by a form of adaptive shortening. In contrast physical training has been found to increase the cross-section area of the muscle fibres with a corresponding increase in muscle bulk and strength (Arvidson et al 1984; Eriksson and Häggmark 1979; Häggmark et al 1981; Thorstensson et al 1977). As noted in (Diez et al 1986), the potential of the adult skeletal muscle fibres to change their biomechanical properties in response to functional demands is indeed remarkable.

An impaired motor drive can also result from lesion and disuse (McComas 1994) and this in turn may be responsible for the reduction in muscle use. Moreover McComas et al (1995) suggest that disuse accentuates muscle fatigue by reducing the ability of the motor centres to recruit motor neurons efficiently. Furthermore a lack of both muscle activity and joint movement results in adaptive anatomical, mechanical, and functional changes to the neural and muscular system, which also leads to a loss of functional motor units (McComas 1994).

According to Carr and Shepherd (2002), this can lead to a change of muscle fibre type, together with a physiological change in the muscle fibre and metabolism, which is evident in a growing sense of stiffness. Muscles thus subjected to a prolonged positioning at a short length, and which are rarely exposed to active and passive stretch, undergo a change in the cross-bridge connection and become shorter (develop contractures) and stiffer (Carr and Shepherd 2002). Changes in the connective tissue also contribute both to stiffness and contracture (William et al 1988), since water loss and collagen deposit also occur as a result of disuse (Carey and Burghardt 1993). An increase in stiffness is also apparent in the absence of contracture (Malouin et al 1997). Clinical and laboratory tests have demonstrated the functional interference caused by increased stiffness (Sinkjaer and Magnussen1994). This reduced activity level in hemiplegic subjects may be responsible for the stress deprivation of muscles, which in turn facilitates the development of muscle stiffness and contracture, all of which serves to compound the difficult task of recovery. Postural muscles with a large proportion of slow twitch fibres (e.g. soleus) may develop stiffness due to a lack of activity, and this stiffness and contracture of the soleus can have importzant functional side-effects by interfering with walking, standing up and balancing in a standing position (Carr and Shepherd 2004)

Prevention of muscle atrophy in hemiplegic subjects:

Carr and Shepherd (2000) suggest that effective motor performance requires that:

- Each muscle should be involved in the generation of peak force at the length appropriate to the action.
- This force has to be graded and timed so that the synergic muscular activity is adapted to the task and context.
- The force has to be sustained over a sufficient period of time.
- The peak force must be generated fast enough to meet environmental task demands such as increasing speed of walking.

Although muscle weakness contributes to the difficulty of performing such functional tasks, muscle strengthening is not alone sufficient for improving functional activity following a stroke.

Task specific training to prevent muscle atrophy in hemiplegic subjects:

Individual muscle strengthening and aerobic exercise are an effective way of improving muscle function. The following discussion will examine the effects of exercise on muscles and assess the appropriateness of task specific training before finally turning to the importance of task repetition for realization of long-term functional improvement.

The neuromuscular ajustment associated with muscle strengthening in the able-bodied is due to an adaptation of the neural drive, which is both quantitative (an increased neural drive to the target muscles) and qualitative (a reduced co-contraction and improved coordination among synergists) (Hakkinen and Komi 1983; Rutherford and Jones 1986; Carolan and Cafarelli 1992; Yue and Cole 1992). The use of various exercises to improve muscle force will enhance their excitation capacity, while at the same time improving the rate of recruitment within the motor neuron pool, the capacity to inhabit agonist muscles, the activation and synchronization of the motor unit, not to mention tuning up the motor firing pattern (Hakkinen and Komi 1983, Sale 1987). More strength training will stimulate metabolic, mechanical and structural muscle fiber changes that result in larger and stronger muscles due to an increase of the actin and myocin protein filaments (Sale 1987; Thepaut-Mathieuet et al 1988). It has been reported that there is a direct correlation between increasing the muscle strength of the lower limbs and an improved standing balance (Bohannon 1988) and walking speed (Sharp and Brouwer 1997, Teixeira-Salmela et al 1999), as well as between the strength of the hand muscles and their functional movements (Butefisch et al 1995). Even so, an increase in strength may not be sufficient to bring about improved walking performance without practice of the action itself, which is essential for the recovery of neural adaptation to the task and context (Rutherford 1988). Thus while strengthening may help to improve force and excitability, as well as operating on the metabolism of the muscles, this may not be sufficient to alter the functional performance of hemiplegic subjects. People with very weak muscles may still be able to improve their functional status to some extent if they practice strengthening exercise.

One of the major problems of therapy is the difficulty in extending the results obtained to other situations beyond that of the therapeutic setting (Hochstenbach and Mulder 1999). During therapy, the context is that of a simplified, protected and predictable hospital environment, while outside patients have to deal with the complex and ever changing world of their surroundings (Hochstenbach and Mulder 1999). Tulving and Thomson (1973) affirm that the more the final application resembles the practice context, the better the retention performance will be. It is thus important for hemiplegic subjects to learn task specific activities in order to change their functional status.

The body adapts specifically to the demands imposed upon it and research over many years has shown that the effects of exercise tend to be related to the task and context (Rutherford1988). Therefore one important strategy is to teach functional tasks, which help to maintain the 'organizational structure' of the muscles. Since motor skills have a specific organizational structure, they should not arbitrarily be broken down for practice (Hochstenbach and Mulder 1999). Here it is further pointed out that a better and more efficient retention will result by preserving the inter-related structure of each sequence of movements. However Buchner et al (1996) have shown that a curvilinear relationship exists between the strength of the lower limbs and walking velocity. They pointed out that this relationship reflects a mechanism by which small changes in strength may produce relatively large changes in performance in the case of very weak adults, while large changes may have little or no effect in-able bodied adults. Therefore when muscles go beyond a certain task-dependent threshold (a threshold that for the majority of everyday tasks is well below normal strength values), exercises are required that are task oriented (Carre Shephard 2004).

Silver and colleagues (2000) have demonstrated the use of an aerobic treadmill training program by a healthy able-bodied person three times a week for three months should result in an increased gait velocity and cadence, together with a decrease in the overall time required to perform a modified 'get up and go' test. Here the exercise intensity was individualized and advanced to 40 minutes' training at approximately 60-70% of maximum heart rate reserve. Moreover Teixera-Salmelda et al (1999) have also tried to evaluate the general physical condition of a subject according to the Human Activity Profile, a survey of ninety four activities, including moving around, home maintenance and participation in social and physical activities, all of which are rated according to their required metabolic equivalents. The results indicated that subjects were more able to perform household chores and recreational activities after strengthening and aerobic training. It is evident that a relationship should exist between strength and function, though the exact nature of this relationship appears complex and is largely dependent on the extent of muscle weakness. Strengthening of individual muscles through exercise or improving the aerobic capacity may not itself have a significant impact on the prevention of muscle atrophy. Still muscular atrophy is attributable to under or reduced activity and therefore a strategy of performing functional tasks seems appropriate as a means of preventing this condition.

Carr and Shepherd (2004) suggest that training involving repetitive practice of the action being learned can in fact improve strength and endurance provided a way is found to increase the load progressively. However Treiber et al (1998) suggest that the conversion of muscle strength into an improved functional performance depends on the ability of subject practicing the task. In both strength training and skill development repetition is an important aspect of practice (Carr and Shepherd 2004). Treiber (1998) has studied tennis players, performing glenohumeral internal and external rotation exercises (incorporating elastic band and hand weight resistance), in a standing position with the shoulder at a 90° abduction. The results showed a significant increase in force production of the actions practiced, which was translated into increased speed of service. Transfer is unlikely to occur, however, unless the subject is already practicing the task to be learned (in the above case, serving in tennis) in some form or another. It is therefore important that hemiplegic subjects learn the functional task and then repeat it in the course of their daily activity. Repetitive practice of the action to be learned can therefore have duel benefits, both enabling the patient to practice the action as well as increasing muscle strength (Rutherford 1988). Moreover, the repetition of functional tasks during the day can facilitate experience-dependent change in the intact neural circuit of the brain, which in turn will ensure a long-term change of functional status in PD subjects.

In conclusion inactivity and under activity is responsible for muscle weakness and atrophy. Studies have demonstrated that a 30% decrease in the force and volume of the quadriceps muscle after one month of immobilisation under a plaster cast. Stroke paralysis results in muscle inactivity, which in turn provokes its atrophy. Muscle weakness can further hinders functional recovery in hemiplegia. Strengthening of individual muscle may prevent its atrophy, though this may not be sufficient to improve functional recovery. It is therefore important that the training program uses task-specific activities.

Bone changes following a stroke:

Introduction: Bone is a specialised type of connective tissue, which supports the structures of the body, protecting the delicate organs such as the heart and lungs and acting as the point of leverage for movement. Stress deprivation resulting from a reduced level of activity may provoke weakness and atrophy of the bone tissue. Moreover the bones of the lower limbs constitute an important organ of locomotion and their atrophy and weakness may be a source of pain and hindrance to the regain of functional autonomy. Therefore it is important to maintain the strength and resilience of the bone tissue. The most striking feature of the bone is that it is the one of the most dynamic and metabolically active tissues of the body, which remains active throughout the course of life (Nordin and Frankel 1994). Here it is further noted that the bone is a highly vascular tissue with an excellent capacity for self-repair and can alter its properties and configuration in response to changes in mechanical demand (Nordin and Frankel 1989). If, on account of a partial or total immobilisation, bone is not subjected to the usual forms of mechanical stress, the periosteal and subperiosteal bone is reabsorbed (Jenkins and Cochran 1969).

Kazarian and Von Gierke (1969) have demonstrated the decreased strength and stiffness of the bone of Rhesus monkey placed in a full-body cast for 60 days. A controlled compression test of the vertebrae from immobilised monkeys conducted in vitro and revealed a threefold decrease in load to failure and the energy storage capacity in the vertebrae concerned and there was also a significant decrease in the toughness of the bone tissue.

<u>Bone atrophy in hemiplegia:</u> Compact and cancellous bone tissue is constantly expanding or contracting in response to the amount of stress placed on them, Dolan (1994). Nordin and Frankel (1989) suggest that the bone has the ability to readjust by altering its size, shape and structure to meet the mechanical demands placed on it. This has been aptly summarised as Wolff's law, which states that 'bone is laid down where needed and reabsorbed where not needed' (Wolff, 1892). A prolonged condition of weightlessness, such as that experienced in space travel, has been found to result in a decreased bone mass of the weight-bearing bones (Rambout and Johnston 1979; Gazenko et al 1981). Moreover greater body weight has been associated with a greater bone mass (Exner et al 1979). This means if a bone is subjected to increased stress its volume also increases. The bones of subjects with hemiplegia may undergo profound structural and mechanical changes, especially if the subject spends much of the day sitting down or laying in the bed. Moreover, since the contraction of the muscles provides added stress on the bone tissue, in hemiplegics muscular paralysis results in the failure to provide this natural stress on the bone tissues.

In addition, this contraction of the muscles serves to transform tensile force on the bone into a compressive force, which further results in a natural toughening of the bone tissue. For example, a contraction of a glutious medius muscle transforms the tensile force on the neck of the femur into a compressive force. However a paralysed glutinous medius muscle may not be able to transform this tensile force during weight bearing into a force of compression. One consequence is that a hemiplegic subject may not be able to perform activities while standing or even maintain themselves in this position and in extreme case the atrophied neck of femur may be fractured as a result of the tensile force during any weight bearing. Thus it would seem that muscular inactivity facilitates the atrophy of the bones, which can be further aggravated if the subject spends much of the day sitting or lying down in bed. Clearly then a reduced level of activity may contribute to the weakness and atrophy of the bone tissue and this can work to impede the regain of functional autonomy.

Factors facilitating bone restructuring

Bone hypertrophy may result if the bone is subjected to repeated mechanical stress within the normal physiological range. Jones et al (1977); Dalén and Olsson (1974); Huddleston et al (1980) have all observed this condition of hypertrophy of normal adult bone tissue in response to strenuous exercise. Nilsson and Westin (1971) have also demonstrated the appearance of an increased bone density after such exercise. Dolan (1994) has argued that during physical exercise such as jogging, the bones are subjected to an increased level of stress and the bone responds accordingly by laying down more collagen fibres and mineral salts to provide for its strengthening. In the case of hemiplegics it is essential to prevent bone atrophy by ensuring constant exercise and by encouraging weight bearing activities.

Degeneration of bone associated with age

Dolan (1995) suggests that in the ongoing process of bone formation and reabsorption, there is a form of balance so that the total amount of tissue does not change. Then from about the age of 35 to 40, the bone tissue begins to be lost as reabsorption exceeds formation (Dolan 1995). According to Nordin and Frankle (1989) a progressive loss of bone density has been observed as part of the normal aging process. Changes of bone density include a thinning of the longitudinal trabeculae and reabsorption of some transverse trabeculae, which result in thinning of the compact bone and a substantial reduction of in the amount of cancellous bone tissue. This thinning of bone tissue markedly reduces the capacity of ther bone to withstand fractures. Burstein et al (1976) studied specimens of human tibia from two subjects of widely differing age, which were tested under stress, and the result showed conclusively that the older bone specimen could withstand only half the strain of the younger, indicating both a condition of brittleness and a reduction in the energy storage capacity. More recently Dolan (1994) has demonstrated that the loss of strength within the bone tissue in older adults is compensated for by changes in the shape of the bone with age. This change manifests itself through the modification in the diameter of the inner and outer bone cortex, where there is an increase in the cross-section area of the bone with age and to a certain extent this would seem to compensate the loss of bone strength.

Conclusion: Bone is a specialised tissue and osteoarthritis is considered as a disease of subchondral bone. Demineralisation, abrasion and micro factures of subchondral bone may cause severe pain. However bone can be remodelled and this may be the key factor in reducing pain and slowing down the progression of the disease. A progressive program of low impact exercises may strengthen the subchondral bone and facilitate a healing of the micro-fractures. Many people with hemiplegia are elderly and here demineralisation as well as reduced fracture toughness is common. This needs to be taken into account when designing a program of progressive exercise.

Change in non-contractile soft tissue

Tendons and ligaments are soft connective tissues, where the tendons connect muscles to bone and ligaments bone to each other (Dolan 1995). Both tendons and ligaments have similar tissue structures and composition, which must be capable of withstanding a very high tensile force (Dolan 1995). In a sedentary position these tendons and ligaments may be subjected to stress deprivation, which can lead to their atrophy and contraction. Inactivity following a stroke may be responsible for structural and functional impairment of these tissues.

The muscles constitute an important structure which provides both stability and mobility of the joints and they form an indispensable organ for the conduct of different functional activities, whereas the tendons and ligaments function as passive stabilisers and thus their weakness and atrophy may aggravate joint instability.

Functionally, tendons and ligaments transmit tensile loads from muscle to bone and allow this to be directed away from the point of action so that bulky bodies do not obstruct any movement (Dolan1995). Ligaments also play a significant role in stabilising the joint, both guiding and limiting its movement. The efficient performance of any of the above functions thus depends greatly on the preservation of the ligaments and tendons in an optimal condition.

Tendons and ligaments both exhibit a form of visco-elasticity or rate-dependent (time-dependent) behaviour, which is to say that they are capable of restructuring to become stronger when subjected to regular stress and weaker when they are deprived of stress. The ligaments are pliant and flexible, allowing for the natural movement of the bones to which they are attached, but at the same time strong and inextensible so as to offer suitable resistance to applied forces (Carlstedt and Nordin 1989). The ligaments and tendons exhibit visco- or fluid-filled elastic behaviour, that is they are subject to 'stress relaxation' (when the tissue is held at a constant length the stress or tension produced by the tissue gradually declines), as well as undergoing 'creep deformation' (when the tendon and ligament extend progressively in response to a constant stretching force). Tendons and ligaments are required to withstand a large tensile force (stretching force), while at the same time they must be flexible enough to wrap around anatomical structures for the joints to move freely (Donal,1994). The tensile property of the ligament depends on its elasticity and varies according to the region of the body. Both the function and structure of ligaments may be subject to change with age. The following discussion examines these behaviours of tendons and ligaments.

A reduced level of activity may be responsible for the deterioration of the structural and functional properties of tendons and ligaments, which include

- Diminution of tensile stress (the capacity to withhold stretching force) and toughness.
- Reduction in the strength of the ligament-bone junction.

Under use of the joints due to a reduced level of activity may be responsible for the acceleration of atrophy in the tendons and ligaments. Still it is not clear just how much activity is required to maintain their mechanical and structural properties in an optimal condition. One theory is that during normal activity, tendons and ligaments are subjected to loads less than a third of that which could occasion injury and these activities are sufficient to maintain their structural and mechanical properties. It is thus essential for hemiplegics actively to engage in repeated forms of activity, while performing weight bearing tasks to minimise the stress deprivation on these tissues.

The changes in ligaments and tendons linked to a reduced level of activity include an increase in the random orientation of the collagen fibres and **a** reduction in the number of cross-links between the collagen molecules. This reduction may extend to as much as 50% after several weeks of immobilisation (Dolan 1994). Moreover biomechanical changes to a ligament after stress deprivation are often accompanied by a contraction (shortening) of the ligament which noticeably increases joint stiffness (Dolan 1994). The author has demonstrated that a ligament of 20 mm in length contracts due to stress deprivation to 19 mm while undergoing a loss of 25% of its other mechanical properties. If, in a certain joint position, this ligament were to be elongated to 20.5 mm, this would mean being subjected to a strain more than three times that of the original ligament. Experiments by Amiel et al (1982) on rabbits that had been immobilised for 9 weeks showed such a decrease in the length and toughness of the lateral collateral ligaments. Since the cross section area of the specimens did not change significantly, the degeneration of the mechanical properties was attributed to changes in the ligament substance itself. The tissue metabolism was observed to increase, which led to the use of proportionally more immature collagen with a corresponding decrease in the number and quality of the cross-links between the collagen molecules.

Dolan (1994) has suggested that even a short period of immobilisation may lead to a rapid and substantial diminution in the structural and mechanical properties of the ligaments, whereas only comparatively small gains are achieved after a period of exercise. An experiment on primates conducted by Noyes (1977), which consisted of an 8-week period of immobilisation follow by recondition training, has demonstrated that considerable time is needed for the immobilised ligaments to regain their former strength and toughness. Even after 5-months the reconditioned ligaments still showed considerably less stiffness and 20% less strength than did ligaments from controlled animals. It was only after a period of 12 months that the reconditioned ligaments had regained a strength and toughness comparable to those of the control group ligaments. Shortened ligaments may be subject to an increased strain rate and this may also be responsible for joint stiffness, which in turn can increase the stress concentration on the articular surface, eventually producing pain in the joint. It is clear then that a reduction in the level of activity in hemiplegic subjects can accelerate the alteration of the structural and mechanical properties of tendons and ligaments leading to their atrophy and shortening. Moreover their altered structural and mechanical properties may provoke joint pain and in extreme case deformity, which may further impede the process of functional recovery. Therefore it is important to maintain the structural and mechanical properties of both tendons and ligaments and prevent their atrophy and shortening. It is easy to provide exercise for different muscles and prevent their stress deprivation. However tendons and ligaments are passive stabilisers and their activation seems more difficult than in the case of muscles. Since the tendons are attached at the end of the muscle, various exercises can help to minimise the stress deprivation of tendons to a certain extent. Due to the fact that the tendons and ligaments function as passive stabilisers, they are mostly brought into action only during weight bearing activities. It is therefore important to start active dynamic exercises from an early stage after a stroke before any deterioration of the structure and functional properties if the tendons and the ligaments can set in. Given that the tendons and ligaments act as the passive stabiliser of the joint during weight bearing activities, so it is essential to perform such activities to provide adequate stress on the tendons and ligaments and to prevent their eventual atrophy.

It can be concluded that ligaments and tendons exhibit a visco- or fluid filled elastic behaviour, that is they are subject to 'stress relaxation' (when the tissue is held at a constant length the stress or tension produced by the tissue gradually declines), as well as undergoing 'creep deformation' (when the tendon and ligament extend progressively in response to a constant stretching force). Tendons and ligaments become stronger and tougher when subjected to increased stress (load per unit area), and weaker in the case of stress deprivation. Various exercises to improve muscle strength can also provide adequate stress on the tendons and ligaments and may therefore contribute to preserve their optimal biomechanical and structural properties. In hemiplegic subjects the stress deprivation resulting from pain and joint underuse may alter the mechanical and structural properties of the tendons and ligaments, which can lead to their growing shorter and this in turn may provoke joint stiffness and pain. With ageing, the collagen content within the tendons and ligaments decreases and this also produces further stress with a diminution of as much as 20% in their stiffness and strength (Dolan 1994).

X

Conclusion

In post-stroke hemiplegia brain damage causes a breakdown of the motor functional architecture. The architectural structure of motor fucntion consists of three distinct systems – program control system, feedback control system, and reflex control system. Maily the program and feedback control system are impaired leaving intact reflex control system. Moreover the reflex control sysem is deprived of the inhibitin and modulating effect from the two other systems. Therefore uninhibted and non-modulated refx activities become the dominating motor activities after a cerebral lesion in hemiplegia. Physical intervention should provide precisely shaped stimulation to restore program and feedback control system of the brain. The chapter on intervention strategy has drawn a wide range research based evidences to identify the precisely shaped stimulation that are effective to restore those two systems. The initial chaper is consecrated the possibility restore different types of neurpalstic activities that can foster in neural circuit of damaged brain. Beside motor impairment congintive impairement is one of the main consequences in lesioned brain. Moreover the cognitive impairement can have interfering effect on the fostering of neuroplaticity. Therefore chapter on cognitive function has described some of the intervention strategies to bypass the interfering effect of cognitive fucntion. Final chapepter has described the secondary consequence on the different musculoskelatal structure in peopla with stroke.

References

Adams J.A. (1971) 'A close-loop theory of motor learning' Journal of Motor Behavour.3, 111-150.

Adams J.A. and Goetz E.T., (1973) 'Feedback and practice as variable in error detection and correction', Journal of Motor Behaviuor. 5, 217-224.

Ada L.and O'Dwyer N (2001) in Carr J; Shepherd R (2004) Stroke rehabilitation, guidelines for exercise and training to optimize motor skill. Elsevier Scientific Limited, London.

Ada I and Westwood P. (1992) in Carr J; Shepherd R (2004) Stroke rehabilitation, guidelines for exercise and training to optimize motor skill. Elsevier Scientific Limited, London.

Allen, C.M.C. (1984). Predicting outcome of acute stroke: a prognostic score. Journal of Neurology, Neurosurgery and psychiatry. 47, 475-80.

Anderson, T.P., Brouestom, N. Hildyard, V.G. (1974) Predictive in stroke rehabilitation. Arch. Phys. Med. Rehibil. Vol 55. P. 545-553.

Anianson A; GrimbyG. Rundgren A. et al (1980) in Carr J; Shepherd R (2004) Stroke rehabilitation, guidelines for exercise and training to optimize motor skill. Elsevier Scientific Limited, London.

Arvidson I, Eriksson E, and Pitman M (1984) 'Neuromuscular basis of rehabilitation. In: Rehabilitation of the injured knee'. Edited by E Hunter and J. Funk. StLouis, C. V. Mosby, P210-234.

Ashburn A. (1997). Physical Recovery Following Stroke. Physiotherapy, September, Vol. 83.No.9.

Ashburn, A and Goodrich, S. (1996) Behavioural deficits associated with the 'pusher syndrome', Proceedings of the World Confederation for Physical Therapy Congress, Washinton, USA.

AsanumaH. And Keller A (1991) in Carr J; Shepherd R (2004) Stroke rehabilitation, guidelines for exercise and training to optimize motor skill. Elsevier Scientific Limited, London.

Batemen A. Culpan F.J. Pickering A.D. et al (2001) in Carr J; Shepherd R (2004) Stroke rehabilitation, guidelines for exercise and training to optimize motor skill. Elsevier Scientific Limited, London.

Bach-y-Rita, P., (1989) Theory-based neurorehabilitation. Arch. Phys. Med.Rehabil. 70, p162

Benecke R, Rothwell J C, Dick JPR, et al (1997) in Morris ME, (2000) Movement Disorder in People with Parkinson Disease: A model for Physical Therapy. Physical Therapy. Volume 80. No 6. P578-597.

Bisiach E. and Vallar G. (1988) in Hochstenbach, J. Mulder, T (1999) Neuropsychology and the relearning of motor skills following stroke. International Journal of Rehabilitation Research. 22. P.11-19.

Bleton, J.P. SteveninP.H. (26451 A10) Rééducation dans le traitement de la maladie de Parkinson. Encycl. Méd. Chir. Paris, Kinésithérapie. 4-4-10.

Bergego, C. Azouvi, P. Deloch, G. Samual, C. Louis-Dreyfus, A Kashel, R. and Williames, K. (1997) Rehabilitation of unilateral neglect: A controlled multiple-baseline across-subjects trial using computerised training procedures. Neuropsychological Rehabilitation, 7. 279-293.

Berger W., Horstmann, G. and Dietz, V. (1984) ,Tension development and muscle activation in spastic hemiparesis: Independence of muscle hypertonia and exaggerated stretch reflex', Journal of Neurology, Neurosurgery and Psychiatry, 47. 1029-33.

Bernstein N. (1967) in Carr J; Shepherd R (2004) Stroke rehabilitation, guidelines for exercise and training to optimize motor skill. Elsevier Scientific Limited, London.

Bobath, B (1991) Adult Hemiplegia: evaluation and Treatment; Butterworth-Heinemann ltd. Oxford.

Brown D.A. Kautz S.A. (1998) in Carr J; Shepherd R (2004) Stroke rehabilitation, guidelines for exercise and training to optimize motor skill. Elsevier Scientific Limited, London.

Bohannon R.W. (1988) in Carr J; Shepherd R Stroke rehabilitation, guidelines for exercise and training to optimize motor skill. Elsevier Scientific Limited, London 2004.

Buchner D.M.Larson E.B. Wagner E.H. (1996) in Carr J; Shepherd R (2004) Stroke rehabilitation, guidelines for exercise and training to optimize motor skill. Elsevier Scientific Limited, London.

Burk, D. (1988) 'Spasticity as an adaptation of pyramidal tract injury' in: waxman, S.G. (ed) Advances in Neurology, 4: Functional recovery in Neurological disease, Raven Press, NewYork, pp401-423.

Burstein A H, Relly D T, Martens M (1976) 'Aging of bone tissue: mechanical properties'. J. Bone Joint Surg., 58A, 82.

Butefisch C. Hummelsheim H. MauritzK.H. (1995) in Carr J; Shepherd R (2004) Stroke rehabilitation, guidelines for exercise and training to optimize motor skill. Elsevier Scientific Limited, London.

Cameron, H.A.et al (1993) 'Differentiation of newly born neurons and galia in the dentate gyrus of the adult rat', Neuroscience 12, 3642-3650.

Canning C.G. Ada L. O4dwyer N.J. (2000) in Carr J; Shepherd R (2004) Stroke rehabilitation, guidelines for exercise and training to optimize motor skill. Elsevier Scientific Limited, London.

Cao, J. Wenberg, K. Cheng, M.F. (2002) Lesion induced new neuron incorporation in the adult hypothalamus of the avian brain. Brain Research. 943; 80-92.

Carey, J.R., and Burghardt, T.P. (1993) 'Movement Dysfunctionfollowing cental nervous system lesion: Aproblem of neurologic or muscular impairment', Physcal Therapy, 73, 538-547.

Carey L.M. Matyas T.A. Oke L.E. et al (1993) in Carr J; Shepherd R (2004) Stroke rehabilitation, guidelines for exercise and training to optimize motor skill. Elsevier Scientific Limited, London.

Carey L.M.(1985) in Carr J; Shepherd R (2004) Stroke rehabilitation, guidelines for exercise and training to optimize motor skill. Elsevier Scientific Limited, London.

Carolan B. And Cafarelli E. (1992) in Carr J; Shepherd R (2004) Stroke rehabilitation, guidelines for exercise and training to optimize motor skill. Elsevier Scientific Limited, London.

Carlstedt and Nordin (1989) in Nordin, M. and Frankel V.H (1989) 'Basic Biomechanics of the Musculoskeletal System'. 2nd edition; Lea and Febiger; Philadelphia, London.

Carter M C and Shapiro D.C. (1984) Control of sequential movements: Evidence for generalised motor programs. Journal of Neuropsychology; Vol.52: p787-796.

Carr J; Shepherd R (2004) Stroke rehabilitation, guidelines for exercise and training to optimize motor skill. Elsevier Scientific Limited, London.

Carr, J.H. Shepherd, R.B. Ada L. (1995) Spasticity: Research findings and Implication for Intervention. Vol. 81. No8.

Chapman, C.E., and Wiessendanger, M (1982) 'The physiological and anatomical basis of spasticity; A review' Physiotherapy Canada, 34, pp125-136.

Colley, A.N. and Beech, J.R. (1988). Grounds for reconciliation: some preliminary thoughts on cognition and action. In cognition and Action in Skilled Behaviour (edited by A.M. Colly and R.J. Beech), PP1-11. Amsterdam.

Cruz –Martinanez A. (1984) in Carr J; Shepherd R (2004) Stroke rehabilitation, guidelines for exercise and training to optimize motor skill. Elsevier Scientific Limited, London. Farmer et al 1993

Dalén N, and Olssen K E (1974) 'Bone mineral content and physical activity'. In : Nordin, M. and Frankel V.H (1989) 'Basic Biomechanics of the Musculoskeletal System' 2nd edition; Lea and Febiger; Philadelphia,

Dellenbourg P. and Schnieder D (1995) School of Psychology and Educational Science, University of Geneva. Switzerland.

Denny-Brown D, and Yanagisawa N (1976) The role of basal ganglia in the initiation of movement. InYahr MD edition, The basal ganglia.Raven Pres, New York.

Dietz, V., Quintern, J. and Berger, W (1981) 'Electrophysiological studies of gait in spasticity and rigidity: Evidence that altered mechanical properties of contribute to hypertonia', Brain, 104, pp431-449.

Dietz, V., Ketelsen, U.P. Berger, W. and Quintern, J (1986) 'Motor unit involvement in spastic paresis: Relationship between leg muscle activation histochemistry', Journal of Neurological Science, 75, 89-103.

Diller, L. and Weinberg, J. (1977). Hemi-inattention in rehabilitation: the evolution of a national remediation program. In Advancces in Neurology (vol. 18) (edited by E.A. Weinstein and R.P. Friedland), pp.63-82. New York: Raven Press.

De Renzi, E and Faglioni, P. Apraxia. In: Denes G.F., Pizzamiglio L. (1999) Handbook of Clinical and Experimental Neuropsychology. Hove: Psychological Press. 421-41.

Darien-Smith I. Galea M.P. Darien-Smith C (1996) in Carr J; Shepherd R (2004) Stroke rehabilitation, guidelines for exercise and training to optimize motor skill. Elsevier Scientific Limited, London.

Dolan M J (1994) 'Skeletal Mechanics'. Orthopaedic and Rehabilitation Technology, Distance Learning Section, Dept of Orthopaedic and Trauma Surgery, University of Dundee, Dundee.

Dolan, M.J. (1995) Tissue Mechanics. Distance Learning Section, Dept of Orthopaedic and Trauma Surgery, University of Dundee, Dundee.

Dong Y, Winstein CJ, Albistegui-DuBois R, Dobkin BH. (2007) Evolution
of fMRI activation in the perilesional primary motor cortex and cerebellum with rehabilitation training-related motor gains after stroke: a pilot study. *Neurorehabil Neural Repair.* 21:p 412-428.

Dong Y, Dobkin BH, Cen SY, Wu AD, Winstein CJ. (2006) Motor cortex activation during treatment may predict therapeutic gains in paretic hand function after stroke. *Stroke.* 37: 1552-1555.

Elbert T., PantevWienbruch cet al (1995), in Carr J; Shepherd R (2004) Stroke rehabilitation, guidelines for exercise and training to optimize motor skill. Elsevier Scientific Limited, London.

Eriksson, P.S. et al (1998) Neurogenesis in the adult human hippocampus Nat.Med.4, 1313-1317.

Exner G U (1979) 'Bone densimetryusing computed tomography. Part I: Selective determination of trabecular bone density and other bone mineral parameters. Normal values in children and adults'. Br. J. Radio., 52 : 14.

Farmer S.F. Swash M. In gram D.A. et al (1993) in Carr J; Shepherd R (2004) Stroke rehabilitation, guidelines for exercise and training to optimize motor skill. Elsevier Scientific Limited, London.

Ericksson E, and Häggmark T (1979) 'Comparison of isometric muscle training and electrical stimulation supplementing isometric muscle training in the recovery after major knee ligament surgery'. Am. J. Sports med., 7 : 169.

Fasotti L and Kovacs F. (1995) in Hochstenbach, J. Mulder, T (1999) Neuropsychology and the relearning of motor skills following stroke. International Journal of Rehabilitation Research. 22. P.11-19.

Feigenson, J.S. McDowell, F.H. Meese, P.D. McCarthy, M.L. Greenberg, S.D. (1977) Factors influencing outcome and length of stay in a stroke rehabilitation unite. Part 1. Analysis of 248 unscreened patients – medical and functional prognosis indicators. Stroke 8: 651-662.

Friel K.M. and Nudo R.J. (1989) in Carr J; Shepherd R (2004) Stroke rehabilitation, guidelines for exercise and training to optimize motor skill. Elsevier Scientific Limited, London.

Galletly R, and Braure S (2005) Does the type of concurrent task affect preferred and cued gait in people with Parkinson's disease? Australian Journal of Physiotherapy. 51: 175-180.

Galski, T. Bruno, R.L. Zorowitz, R. Walker, J. (1993) Predicting length of stay, functional outcome, and aftercare in the rehabilitation of stroke patients. The dominant role of higher order of cognition. Stroke 24. 1794-1800.

Gazenko O G, Genin A M, and Yegrov A D (1981) In : Nordin, M. and Frankel V.H (1989) 'Basic Biomechanics of the Musculoskeletal System' 2nd edition; Lea and Febiger; Philadelphia, London.

Goldberg G. (1995) 'Imitating of gestures and manipulating a mannik in the representation of the human body in idiomotor apraxia', Neuropsychologia 33, 63-72.

Gould, E., Tanapat, P., Hastings, N.B., Shors, T.J. (1999) Neurogenesis in adulthood: a possible in learning. Trend in Cognitive Sciences – Vol. 3. P. 186 – 192.

Gould, E. et al (1997) 'Neurogenesis in the dentate gyrus of the adult tree shrew is regulated by psychological stress and NMDA receptor activation', Journal of Neuroscences.17. 2492-2498.

Häggmark T, Jansson E, and Eriksson E (1981) 'Fibre type area and metabolic potential of the thigh muscle in man after knee surgery and immobilisation'. Int. J. Sports Med. 2 : 12.

Hakkinen K. And Komi P.V. (1983) in Carr J; Shepherd R Stroke rehabilitation, guidelines for exercise and training to optimize motor skill. Elsevier Scientific Limited, London 2004.

Halkjear-Kristenson J, and Ingemann-Hansen T (1985) 'Wasting of the human quadriceps muscle after knee ligament injuries. 1. Anthropometric consequences'. Scandanavian Journal of Rehabil Med Suppl, 13, P5-55.

Halligan P.W. Cokburn J. Wilson B.A. (1991) in Hochstenbach, J. Mulder, T (1999) Neuropsychology and the relearning of motor skills following stroke. International Journal of Rehabilitation Research. 22. P.11-19.

Harris, J.E., and Sanderland, A. (1981). A brief survey of the management of memory disorders in rehabilitation units in Britain. International Rehailitation Medicine, 3, 206-209.

Heilman, M.K. and Ven Den Abell, T. (1997) Right hemisphre dominancefor mediating cerebral activation. Neuropsychologia, 17, 315-321.

Hochstenbach, J. Mulder, T (1999) Neuropsychology and the relearning of motor skills following stroke. International Journal of Rehabilitation Research. 22. P.11-19.

Holden A, Wilman A, Wieler M, Martin W (2006) Basal ganglia activation in Parkinson's disease, Parkinsonism related disorder. 12:73-77.

Hollis M. (1988) Practical Exercise Therapy. Blackwell Scientific Publication, UK

Hom, J. and Reitan, R.M. (1990). Generalised cognitive function after stroke. Journal of clinical and experimental Neuropsychology, 12, 644-654.

Huddleston A L, Rockwell D, Kuluund D N, and Harrison R B (1980) 'Bone mass in lifetime tennis athletes.' JAMA, 244, P1107-1109.

Hufschimdt, A. and Mauritz K.H (1985) 'Chronic transformation of muscle in spasticity: a peripheral contribution to increased tone', Journal of Neurology, Neurosurgery and Psychiatry, 48, 676-685.

Hummelsheim H. Munch B. Butefisch C et al (1994) in Carr J; Shepherd R) Stroke rehabilitation, guidelines for exercise and training to optimize motor skill. Elsevier Scientific Limited, London 2004.

Hyvarinen J. Poranen A. Jokinen Y. (1980) In Carr J; Shepherd R (2004) Stroke rehabilitation, guidelines for exercise and training to optimize motor skill. Elsevier Scientific Limited, London.

Ietswaart, M., Carey, D.P., Della Salla, S., Dijkhuizen. R.F. 2001) Memory-drivenovements in limb apraxia: is there evidence for impaired communication between the dorsal and the ventral streams?

Jenkins W.M. Merzenich M.M. Ochs M.T. et al (1990) in Carr J; Shepherd R Stroke rehabilitation, guidelines for exercise and training to optimize motor skill. Elsevier Scientific Limited, London 2004.

Jenkins D P, and Cochran T H (1996) 'Osteoporosis; dynamic effect of disuse of an extremity.' in Nordin, M. and Frankel V H (1989) 'Basic Biomechanics of the Musculoskeletal System' 2nd edition; Lea and Febiger; Philadelphia, London.

Jones H H, et al (1977) 'Humeral hypertrophy in response to exercise'. In : Nordin, M. and Frankel V.H (1989)'Basic Biomechanics of the Musculoskeletal System' 2nd edition; Lea and Febiger; Philadelphia, London.

Jueptener M, Frith C, Brook D et al (1997) Subcortical structures and learning by trial and error. Journal of Neurophysiology. 77: 1325-1337.

Kalra, L. et la (1997) The influence of visual neglect on stroke rehabilitation. Stroke. 28, 1386-1391.

Kampermann, Brandon, E.P., Gage, F.H. (1998) Environmental stimulation of 129/Svj mice caused increased cell proliferation and neurogenesis in the adult dentate gyrus. Curr. Biol. 8, 939-942.

Kampermann, G. Kuhn, H.G., Gage, F.H. (1997) More hippocampal neurones in adult mice living in an enriched environment. Nature 386, 493-49

Katz, R.T. and Rymer, Z. (1989) Spastic Hypertonia: Mechanism and Measurement. Archive of Physical Medicine and Rehabilitation. Vol. 70. P144 –155.

Kautz S.A. and Brown D.A (1989) in Carr J; Shepherd R (2004) Stroke rehabilitation, guidelines for exercise and training to optimize motor skill. Elsevier Scientific Limited, London.

Kazarian L E, and Von Gierke H E (1969) 'Bone loss as a result of immobilisation and chelation. Preliminary results in Macaca mulatta.' Clin. Orthop., 65, P67-75.

Keele S.W. and Posner M.(1986) 'Processing of feedback in rapid movements', Journal of Experimental Psychology. 77,155-158.

Klapp H.E. (1975) in Mak M.K.Y, and Cole J.H, (1991) Movement dysfunction in patient with Parkinson's disease: A literature review; Australian Physiotherapy; Vol.37, no.1, 1991. 7-17.

Kokotilo K.J., Eng J.J., McKeown M.J., LA Boyd L.A., Greater Activation of Secondary Motor Areas Is Related to Less Arm Use

After Stroke. Neurorehabilitation and Neural Repair 2010, 24(1) 78-87.

Kuhn, H.G., Dickson-Anson, H. Gage, F.H.(1996) Neurogenesis in the denetate gyrus of the adult rat: age related decrease of the neuronal progenitor proliferation. Journal of neurosciences, 16, 2027-2023.

Luria, A.L. et al. (1975) 'Restoration of higher cortical functions following local brain damage.' Handbook of clinical of clinical neurology (Vol. 3) (Vinken, P.J.and BrruynG.W. eds). Page 368-499.

Lance J.M. (1980) in Carr J; Shepherd R (2004) Stroke rehabilitation, guidelines for exercise and training to optimize motor skill. Elsevier Scientific Limited, London.

Landau, W.M. (1980) 'Spasticity: Whatis it? What is not?' in: Feldman, R.G. Young, R.R. and Koella, W.P. (eds) Spasticity: Disordered motor control, Year Book of Medical Publishers, Chicago, pp17-24.

Landau, W. M. (1988) Parables of palsy, pills and PT pedagogy: A spastic dialectic. Neurology. 38. P1496 – 99.

Ladavas E et al (1997) in Robertson. I.H. (1999) Cognitive rehabilitation: Attention and neglect. Trend in Cognitive Sciences – Vol. 3. No. 10.

Lee R.G. and Van Do, kelaar P. (1999) in Luria, A.L. et al. (1975) 'Restoration of higher cortical functions following local brain damage.' Handbook of clinical of clinical neurology (Vol. 3) (Vinken, P.J.and BrruynG.W. eds). Page 368-499.

Lee D.N. Aronson E (1974) in Carr J; Shepherd R (2004) Stroke rehabilitation, guidelines for exercise and training to optimize motor skill. Elsevier Scientific Limited, London.

Lewis S JG; Dove A; Robbins TW, Barker RJ; Owen AM; (2003) Cognitive Impairments in Early Parkinson's Disease Are Accompanied By Reduction in Activity in Frontostriatal Neural Circuitry. The Journal of Neuroscienc, July, 23(15 P6351 – 6356.

Lezak, M. (1995). Neuropsychological assessment. New York: Oxford University Press.

Lezak, M.D. (1982) The problem of assessing executive functions. International Jurnal of Psychology. 39, 592-8.

Lincoln, N. Blackburn, M. Ellis, S. Jackson, J. Edmans, J. Nuri. F. and Hawarth, H. (1989) An investigation of factors affecting progress of patients on stroke unit. Journal of Neurology, Neurosurgery and Psychiatry, 52, p493 – 493.

Lindboe C F, and PLatou C S (1984) 'Effect of immobilization of short duration on the muscle fibre size'. Clin. Physiol., 4, P183-188.

Lipert J., Tegenthoff M., Malin J.P. (1995) in Carr J; Shepherd R (2004) Stroke rehabilitation, guidelines for exercise and training to optimize motor skill. Elsevier Scientific Limited, London.

Lovely, R.G., Gregor, R.J., Roy, R.R., Edgerton, V.R. (186) 'Effects of training nthe recovery of full-weight bearing stepping in the adult spinal cat', Experimental Neurology, 92, 421-435.

Luria, A.L. et al. (1975) 'Restoration of higher cortical functions following local brain damage.' Handbook of clinical of clinical neurology (Vol. 3) (Vinken, P.J.and BrruynG.W. eds). Page 368-499.

Luria (1973) The working brain. Penguin press, London.

MACKinnon C.D. Winter D.A. (1993) in Carr J; Shepherd R (2004) Stroke rehabilitation, guidelines for exercise and training to optimize motor skill. Elsevier Scientific Limited, London.

Magill, M.D. (1993). Motor learning: Concept and Application. Madison: WCB.

Majsak MJ, Kaminski T, Gentile AM, Flanagan RJ, (1998) 'The reaching movements of patients with Parkinson's disease under self-determined maximal speed and visually cued conditions.' Brain121(pt 4), P755-766.

Mak M.K.Y, Cole J.H, (1991) Movement dysfunction in patient with Parkinson's disease: A literature review; Australian Physiotherapy; Vol.37, no.1, 1991. 7-17.

Malouin, F, Povtin, M. Prevost, J. Richards, C.L. and Wood-Dauphnee, S. (1992), 'use of intensive task-oriented gait training program in series of patients with acute cerebrovascular accidents', Physical Therapy, 72 pp781-793.

McComas A.J. (1994) in Carr J; Shepherd R (2004) Stroke rehabilitation, guidelines for exercise and training to optimize motor skill. Elsevier Scientific Limited, London.

McComas A.J. Miller R.J. Gandevia S.G. (1995) in Carr J; Shepherd R (2004) Stroke rehabilitation, guidelines for exercise and training to optimize motor skill. Elsevier Scientific Limited, London.

Miller G.J.K. and Light K.E. (1997) in Carr J; Shepherd R (2004) Stroke rehabilitation, guidelines for exercise and training to optimize motor skill. Elsevier Scientific Limited, London.

Milner A.D. (1989) in Robertson. I.H. (1999) Cognitive rehabilitation: Attention and neglect. Trend in Cognitive Sciences – Vol. 3. No. 10.

Milner A.D.and Goodale M.A (1995) in Robertson. I.H. (1999) Cognitive rehabilitation: Attention and neglect. Trend in Cognitive Sciences – Vol. 3. No. 10.

Morris M E, (2005) Impairments, activity limitation and participation restriction in Parkinson's disease. In: Refshauge K, Ada L, Ellis eds. Science based Rehabilitation: Theories into practice. London, UK, Butterworth Heinemann ; 223-248.

Morris ME, (2000) Movement Disorder in People with Parkinson Disease: A model for Physical Therapy. Physical Therapy. Volume 80. No 6. P578-597.

Morris M E, and Iansek R (1997) 'Gait disorder in Parkinson's disease: a framework for physical therapy practice' Neural Rep. 21: P125-131.

Morris ME, Collier J, Matyas TA, et al (1998) Evidence for motor skill learning in Parkinson's disease. In PiekJ. Ed Motor Behaviour and Human Skill: A multidisciplinary approach Champaign, III: Human Kinetics Inc, 329-354.

Nathan P.W. (1980) in Bobath, B (1991) Adult Hemiplegia: evaluation and Treatment; Butterworth-Heinemann ltd. Oxford.

Nelles G. Jentzen W. Jueptner M. et al (2001) Carr J; Shepherd R (2004) Stroke rehabilitation, guidelines for exercise and training to optimize motor skill. Elsevier Scientific Limited, London.

Nordin M and Frankel V H (1989) 'Basic Biomechanics of the Musculoskeletal System' 2nd edition; Lea and Febiger; Philadelphia, London.

Novack, T.A., Huban, G. Graham, K. and Satterfield, W.T. (1987) Prediction of stroke rehabilitation outcome from psychological screening. Archives of Physical Medicine and rehabilitation.68. 729-34.

Noyes F R (1977) 'Functional properties of Knee Ligaments and aleration induced by immobilisation'. Clin.Orthop. 123 : 210.

Nudo R.J. (2003) Adaptive Plasticity in Motor Cortex : Implication for Rehabilitationn after brain injury. J. Rehab. Med., Sup. 41, p7-10.

Nudo R.J Plautz E.J. Frost S.B. (2001) in Carr J; Shepherd R (2004) Stroke rehabilitation, guidelines for exercise and training to optimize motor skill. Elsevier Scientific Limited, London 2004.

Nudo, R.J. et al (1996) in Robertson. I.H. (1999) Cognitive rehabilitation: Attention and neglect. Trend in Cognitive Sciences – Vol. 3. No. 10.

Otis J.C. RRoot I KrollM.A. (1985) in Carr J; Shepherd R) Stroke rehabilitation, guidelines for exercise and training to optimize motor skill. Elsevier Scientific Limited, London 2004.

Pai Y. and Roger M.W. (1990) in Carr J; Shepherd R (2004) Stroke rehabilitation, guidelines for exercise and training to optimize motor skill. Elsevier Scientific Limited, London.

Pascual-Leone A., and Torres F., (1993) in Carr J; Shepherd R (2004) Stroke rehabilitation, guidelines for exercise and training to optimize motor skill. Elsevier Scientific Limited, London.

Pascual-leone A, Wassermann E.M., Sadato N., et al (1993) in Carr J; Shepherd R (2004) Stroke rehabilitation, guidelines for exercise and training to optimize motor skill. Elsevier Scientific Limited, London.

Perry, J. (1980) Rehabilitation of spasticity' in: Feldman ; R.G., Young, R.R. and Koella, W.P. (ed.) Spasticity: Disordered motor control, Year Book of Medical Publishers, Chicago, pp 87- 100.

Plautz E.J. Milliken G.W. NudoR.J. (200) in Nudo R.J. (2003) Adaptive Plasticity in Motor Cortex : Implication for Rehabilitationn after brain injury. J. Rehab. Med., Sup. 41, p7-10.

Prigatano, G.P. (1988). Emotion and motivation in recovery and adaptation after brain damage. In Brin Injury and Recovery. Theoretical and controversial issues (edited by S.Finger, T.E. Levere, C.R. Almli and D.G. Stein), pp335-50. New York: Plenum Press.

Proctor, R. W. and Dutta, A. (1995) Skill Acquisition and Human Performance. London: sage publication.

Rambaut P C and Johnston R S (1979) 'Prolonged weightlessness and calcium loss in man.' Acta Astotronautica, 6 : 1113- 1117

Recanzone, G.H., Schreiner, C. E. and Merzeinch, M. M. (1993) Plasticity in the frequency representation of primary auditory cortex following Discrimination Training in Adult Owl Monkeys. The Journal of Neuroscience. 13(1). 87-103.

Rizzolati G. An Camarda R (1987) in Robertson. I.H. (1999) Cognitive rehabilitation: Attention and neglect. Trend in Cognitive Sciences – Vol. 3. No. 10.

Robertson I.H.and Marshall J.C. (1993) in Robertson. I.H. (1999) Cognitive rehabilitation: Attention and neglect. Trend in Cognitive Sciences – Vol. 3. No. 10.

Robertson. I.H, Hogg, K. and Mcmillan, T.M. (1998) 'Rehabilitation of Unilateral Neglect: Improving Function by Contalesional Limb Activation', Neuropsychological Rehabilitation. 8 (1) 19-29.

Robertson. I.H. (1999) Cognitive rehabilitation: Attention and neglect. Trend in Cognitive Sciences – Vol. 3. No. 10.

Robertson I.H. Nico D. and Hood B.M. (1997) in Robertson. I.H. (1999) Cognitive rehabilitation: Attention and neglect. Trend in Cognitive Sciences – Vol. 3. No. 10.

Robertson I.J. AND Murrre J.M. J (1999) in Robertson. I.H. (1999) Cognitive rehabilitation: Attention and neglect. Trend in Cognitive Sciences – Vol. 3. No. 10.

Reding, M.J.; Gardener, C., Hainline, B. (1993) Neuropsychiatric problems interfering with inpatient stroke rehabilitation. Journal of Neurological Rehabilitation. 7, 1-7.

Rutherford O.M. (1988) in Carr J. Shepherd R Stroke rehabilitation, guidelines for exercise and training to optimize motor skill. Elsevier Scientific Limited, London 2004.

Rutherford O.M. and Jones D.A. (1994) in Carr J. Shepherd R Stroke rehabilitation, guidelines for exercise and training to optimize motor skill. Elsevier Scientific Limited, London 2004.

Sahrmann, S.A. and Norton, B.S. (1977) 'The relationship of voluntary movement to spasticity in the upper motor neuron syndrome', Annals of Neurology, 2, 460-465.

Sale D.G. (1987) in Carr J; Shepherd R Stroke rehabilitation, guidelines for exercise and training to optimize motor skill. Elsevier Scientific Limited, London 2004.

Schmidt (1982) in Mak M.K.Y, and Cole J.H. Movement dysfunction in patient with Parkinson's disease: A literature review; Australian Physiotherapy. 1991, Vol.37, no.1, 7-17.

Schenkman M; Berger R.A. O'Riley P. (1990) in Carr J; Shepherd R (2004) Stroke rehabilitation, guidelines for exercise and training to optimize motor skill. Elsevier Scientific Limited, London.

Schmidt R.A. (1980) in Mak M.K.Y, and Cole J.H. Movement dysfunction in patient with Parkinson's disease: A literature review; Australian Physiotherapy. 1991, Vol.37, no.1, 7-17.

Schmidt R.A.(1976) in Mak M.K.Y, and Cole J.H. Movement dysfunction in patient with Parkinson's disease: A literature review; Australian Physiotherapy. 1991, Vol.37, no.1, 7-17.

Schmidt R.A. and RusselD.G. (1972) Movement Velocity and movement time as determiners of the degree of preprogramming in simple movements' Journal of Experimental Psychology 96. 315-320.

Schultz W, Apilcella P, Romo R, Scarnati E (1995) 'Contex-dependent activity in primate striatum reflecting past and future behavioral events'. In: Houk JC, Devis JL, Beiser DC, edsModels of information processing in the basal ganglia. Cambridge, Mass: P11-27.

Seitz, R.J. et al (1995) Large-scale plasticity of the human motor cortex; Neuro Report 6, p742-744.

Sharp S.A. and Bower B.J. (1997) in Carr J; Shepherd R (2004) Stroke rehabilitation, guidelines for exercise and training to optimize motor skill. Elsevier Scientific Limited, London.

Shepherd R.B.and Gentile A.M. (1994) in Carr J; Shepherd R (2004) Stroke rehabilitation, guidelines for exercise and training to optimize motor skill. Elsevier Scientific Limited, London.

Sinkjaer TMagnussen I. (1994) in Carr J; Shepherd R (2004) Stroke rehabilitation, guidelines for exercise and training to optimize motor skill. Elsevier Scientific Limited, London.

SmithG.V. Macko R.F. SilverK.H.C. et al (1999) in Carr J; Shepherd R. (2004) Stroke rehabilitation, guidelines for exercise and training to optimize motor skill. Elsevier Scientific Limited, London 2004.

Spires TL, and Hannan AJ, (2005) Nature, nurture and neurology: gene-environment interaction in neurodegenerative disease. FEBS Journal. 272: 2347-2361.

prague J.M. (1966) Robertson. I.H. (1999) Cognitive rehabilitation: Attention and neglect.

Trend in Cognitive Sciences – Vol. 3. No. 10.

Squire, L.R., Odo, L.R., Knowlton, B. and MUsen, G., (1993). The structure and organization of memory. Annual review of psychology, 44, 439-95.

Sundet, K. Finset, A. Reinvang, I (1988) Neuropsychological predictors in stroke rehabilitation. Journal of clinical and experimental neuropsychology, 10, 363-79.

Sutherland D. A. Kaufman K.R. Moitoza J.R. (1994) in Carr J; Shepherd R (2004) Stroke rehabilitation, guidelines for exercise and training to optimize motor skill. Elsevier Scientific Limited, London.

Tatemichi, T.K. Desmond, D.W. Stern, Y. Paik. M. Sano, M. and Bageilla, E. (1994) Cognitive impairment after stroke: Frequency, patterns, and relationship to functional abilities. Journal of Neurology, Neurosurgery and Psychiatry, 57, 202-7.

Taub, E (1980) 'Somatosensory deafferentation research with monkeys: Implication for rehabilitation medicine' In: Ince, L.P. (ed) Behavioral Psychology in Rehabilitation Medicine: Clinical applications, Willams and Wilkins, Baltimore, pp 371-401.

Teixera-Salmela L.F. Olney S.J. Nadeau S. et al (1999) in Carr J; Shepherd R (2004) Stroke rehabilitation, guidelines for exercise and training to optimize motor skill. Elsevier Scientific Limited, London.

Thepaut-Mathieu C. Van Hoecke J. MatonB. (1988) in Carr J; Shepherd R Stroke rehabilitation, guidelines for exercise and training to optimize motor skill. Elsevier Scientific Limited, London 2004.

Thorstensson A, Larsson L, Tesch P, and Karlsson J (1977) 'Muscle strength and fibre composition in athletes and sedentary men'. Med. Sc. Sports, 9 : 26.

Tinetti M.F. Speechely M. Ginter S.F. (1988) in Carr J; Shepherd R (2004) Stroke rehabilitation, guidelines for exercise and training to optimize motor skill. Elsevier Scientific Limited, London.

Travis, A.M. and Woolsey, C.W. (1956) 'Motor Performance of monkeys after bilateral, partial and total cerebral decortications' American Journal of Physical Medicine, 35, pp273-310.

Treiber F.A. LottJ. Duncan J.et al (1998) in Carr J; Shepherd R (2004) Stroke rehabilitation, guidelines for exercise and training to optimize motor skill. Elsevier Scientific Limited, London.

Tulving, E. (1972). Episodic and semantic memory. In: Organisation of Memory (edited by E. tulving and W. Donalddson), pp. 381-403. New York: Academic Press.

Tulving E. and Thomson D.M. (1973) in Hochstenbach, J. Mulder, T (1999) Neuropsychology and the relearning of motor skills following stroke. International Journal of Rehabilitation Research. 22. P.11-19.

Valler, G. (1998) Spatial hemineglect in humans. Trends in Cognitive sciences. Vol. 2. 87-97.

Valler, G. (1993) The basis of spatial neglect inhumans, in Unilateral neglect: Clinical and Experimental studies (Robertson, I.H. and Marshalll, J.C. eds) pp27-59, Erlbaum.

Visintin,. M. and Barbeau, H. (1989) 'The effect of body weight support on the locomotion pattern of spastic paretic patients', Canadian Journal of Neurological Sciences, 16, 315-325.

Waddington P.J. (1989) in Hollis M. (1989) Practical Exercise Therapy. Blackwell Scientific Publication, UK

Wagenaar (1990) in Carr J; Shepherd R Stroke rehabilitation, guidelines for exercise and training to optimize motor skill. Elsevier Scientific Limited, London 2004.

Wagenaar R.C. and BeekW.J. (1992) in Carr J; Shepherd R Stroke rehabilitation, guidelines for exercise and training to optimize motor skill. Elsevier Scientific Limited, London 2004.

Walshe F.M.R. (1923) in Bobath, B (1991) Adult Hemiplegia: evaluation and Treatment; Butterworth-Heinemann ltd. Oxford.

Ward NS, Brown MM, Thompson AJ, Frackowiak RS. (2003)Neural correlates of outcome after stroke: a cross-sectional fMRI study. *Brain*. 126: P1430-1448.

Williams P.E. Catanese T. Lucey E.G. (1988) in Carr J; Shepherd R Stroke rehabilitation, guidelines for exercise and training to optimize motor skill. Elsevier Scientific Limited, London 2004.

Winter D.A. (1987) in Carr J; Shepherd R (2004) Stroke rehabilitation, guidelines for exercise and training to optimize motor skill. Elsevier Scientific Limited, London.

Winter D.A. Patla A.E. Frank J.S. et al (1990) in Carr J; Shepherd R (2004) Stroke rehabilitation, guidelines for exercise and training to optimize motor skill. Elsevier Scientific Limited, London.

Wolff (1892) in Dolan M J (1994) 'Skeletal Mechanics'. Orthopaedic and Rehabilitation Technology, Distance Learning Section, Dept of Orthopaedic and Trauma Surgery, University of Dundee, Dundee.

Woodlee M.T., Schallert T., (2004) The interplay between behavior and neurodenegeneration in rat models of Parkinson's disease and stroke. Restor Neural and Neurosci. Vol.22 p153-161.

Yekutel M. and Guttman E. (1993) in Carr J. Shepherd R. (2004) Stroke rehabilitation, guidelines for exercise and training to optimize motor skill. Elsevier Scientific Limited, London.

Yue G. And Cole K.J. (1992) in Carr J. Shepherd R. (2004) Stroke rehabilitation, guidelines for exercise and training to optimize motor skill. Elsevier Scientific Limited, London.

Zmeren, Van, A.H. and Brouwer, W.H., (1994). Clinical Neuropsychology of Attention. NewYork: Oxford University Press.

A GUIDE TO UPHOLD PHYSICAL ACTIVITY LEVEL IN PEOPLE WITH PARKINSON'S DISEASE

I

Introduction

Parkinson's disease (PD) is a specific deficit of transmitter metabolism within the basal ganglia (BG) neurons of the brain and their connections. Greenfield and Bosanquet (1953) state that due to a progressive loss of substantia nigra neurons that produce dopamine, a neurotransmitter imbalance occurs in the basal ganglia. Neurotransmitter imbalance disrupts the function of basal ganglia and their connections. This functional disruption within the BG in turn produces a wide range of motor, cognitive, and behaviour dysfunctions in PD. Given that the BG neurons have wide range of connections with the different areas of the brain, the predominant PD symptoms depend on the area of the BG, and the connections that are most affected. For this reason two PD subjects do not present with similar symptoms. However many PD subjects present with motor dysfunction and require physical rehabilitation intervention in order to uphold their motor function and physical activity level. Motor symptoms include tremor at rest, rigidity of muscle and a difficulty to generate organise kinematic motor activity to perform different functional tasks. This difficulty to generate kinematic motor organisation is mainly due to an impaired program controlled system of the brain. Program controlled system of the brain involves in storing and retrieving of learned motor activities. In order to perform functional tasks the previously learned motor activities are retrieved spontaneously as a chain of interrelated and mutually dependent activities of multiple muscles. Moreover these retrieved muscle activities have specific organisational structure and are specific for each functional task (detailed description is made in the chapter on program control system). BG neurons and their connections play an important role in the generation of program controlled muscle activities, and the neurotransmitter imbalance within BG is responsible for the progressive difficulty in spontaneously retrieving of those activities. In a large number of people with PD, the movement dysfunction is a retrieving difficulty of pre-programmed motor activities, leading to a difficulty to perform different functional tasks. The tasks difficulties in turn contribute to the progressive decline of autonomy and eventual development of functional disabilities in many PD subjects. Therefore the movement strategies which can minimise the difficulty to perform different functional task can help PD subjects to uphold functional activity level and prevent the development of disability. Given that the BG neurons and their connections mediate not only motor function but also different cognitive and behaviour function, and therefore the presence of those associated dysfunctions can aggravate the difficulty to perform motor function and the process of declining autonomy. This chapter encompasses the underlying factors of kinematic motor dysfunction, and the possible strategies to uphold functional activity level in PD subjects.

The chapter on anatomy will review some basic anatomy of the BG, given that the dysfunction of BG and their connections is responsible for the difficulty to retrieve spontaneously pre-program motor activities. This chapter include different nuclei of BG, their connections within themselves as well as with other motor areas are also discussed.

It is essential to understand the function of BG, which can give more insights regarding the consequences of their dysfunction. The focus of the discussion is made to highlight the role of BG as an important part functional architecture that mediates kinematic motor organisation. The role of BG as a storing and retrieving unit of the previously learned movements of the brain is also reviewed. The discussion also highlights the role of dopamine in proper functioning of the BG.

The chapter on the diagnosis of PD has mainly examined the difference between PD and other brain impairments which produce similar symptoms as PD. Early dementia can produce similar symptoms as

Besides the cognitive and behavioural dysfunction, one of the principal attributes for the progressive decline of activity level in PD subjects is disruption in the process of kinematic motor organisation. The dopamine metabolism defect disrupts the structure of functional architecture that mediates motor activities. Precisely the program control system within the motor functional architecture is impaired, which in turn produce four distinct movement dysfunctions. Moreover these four movement dysfunctions are responsible for the progressive decline of autonomy and the development of disability. Because these dysfunctions constitute the underlying factors for the difficulty to initiate, adapt, and readapt within the environment during performing functional tasks. The chapter on the repercussion of defective neurotransmitter metabolism on motor function has highlighted the fact that an impaired program controlled muscle activities

The declined activity level in large number of PD subjects is mainly due to these four distinct movement dysfunctions. Therefore the movement strategies that minimise these dysfunctions are discussed.

Given that the storing and retrieving of learned motor activities are mediated by the BG; and their dysfunction results in an impairment of spontaneous execution of learned movements. Motor activities are learned and stored as motor programs, which can be retrieved as a whole program. These programmed activities largely mediate the kinematic organisation of muscle activities during functional tasks, PD results in an impairment of kinematic organisation of muscle activities, which can eventually be responsible for the progressive difficulty in performing functional task. Therefore the chapter has reviewed some of the insights of these four major movement dysfunctions, their repercussion on the performance of functional tasks at home.

Some movement strategies can help PD subjects to minimise those four movement and eventually help them to uphold their functional activity level. Therefore a detailed description is made on the different movement strategies that can be adapted to minimise each of those four movement dysfunctions.

Moreover the neurotransmitter dysfunction in the BG may produce other symptoms like rigidity of muscles and tremor at rest.

Basal ganglia are also involved in the mediation behaviours unrelated to movements and play a role in different cognitive activities (Côté and Crutcher 1991). Therefore the neurotransmitter metabolism dysfunction in BG is not only responsible for the breakdown of kinematic organisation of muscle activities but also there can be a wide range of cognitive and behaviour dysfunction. The dysfunction of automatic execution of learned motor activities in turn can be responsible for the difficulty to perform different tasks of daily living like getting in and out of the bed getting in and out of a chair, and moving around within a confined space. These task difficulties along with impaired cognitive function can be responsible for the progressive development of disability in many PD subjects. This chapter on Parkinson rehabilitation strategy mainly deal with the movement strategy to ease the difficulty to perform the functional tasks at home, which can slow the development of disabling process.

Moreover the difficulty of task performance is responsible for the progressive decline of autonomy and the development of disability in many PD subjects. In contrast minimising task difficulties may slow the decline of autonomy and hinder the progression of disabling process. However BG degeneration not only limit to motor dysfunction but there can also be wide range of cognitive and behavior dysfunctions. Bhatia and Marsden (1994) affirm that sensory, emotional, and perceptual signs are observed in some individuals. Resting tremor, rigidity and, later in the disease process, postural instability and falls are characteristic of PD. These associated dysfunctions also contribute to the difficulty to perform functional task and eventual development of disability.

As mentioned that the BG are responsible for that automatic execution of learned movements, however movement analysis in PD subjects reveal that several underlying movement dysfunctions, which are hindering factors for the tasks of daily living. These movement dysfunctions include - absence of spontaneous background movements, - difficulty to initiate and execute movements, - difficulty to perform large amplitude movements, - and finally extra difficulty in executing simultaneous and composite movements. However some of these movement dysfunctions can be minimised if PD subjects can use an alternative movement strategy. The alternative movement strategies include the use of conscious voluntary movements and external sensory cues, as well as disintegrate complex movements into several simple movements. Most striking is that these strategies generate movement by bypassing the involvement of BG, which is an important consideration. Since PD is a degenerative disease and people with this disease will be less and less reliant on the BG function, and it is important to exploit the other motor areas to perform different functional task. It can be assumed that PD subjects without severe cognitive and behaviour dysfunction may be able to reduce the difficulty to perform three functional tasks at home by adapting the alternative movement strategies, which bypasses the involvement of BG. However there is no research based evidence to support that the people with PD can integrate an alternative movement strategy to ease the difficulty to perform three functional tasks at home. Therefore, it seems essential to undertake a study to investigate the possibility to ease the difficulty to perform three functional tasks at home and its impact on the activity level in people with PD.

Reduced activity level can be responsible for the weakness and atrophy of different contractile and non contractile tissues, which include bone, muscles tendons, ligaments and cartilage. The atrophy these tissues followed by an adaptive change, which include shortening of different contractile and non contractile tissues, and reduced bone and cartilage density. These adaptive changes of different tissues can further aggravate the difficulty to perform functional tasks at home. Unfortunately strengthening exercise to improve the structure and function of these tissues may not ease the difficulty of task performance because the underlying cause for the difficulty to perform function is linked to defective BG function. Therefore strengthening exercises program, aerobic exercise, treadmill walking, and group gymnastic may have little or no impact on functional status of PD subjects. However Scandalis et al (2001) suggest that progressive resistance strengthening training has been shown to have beneficial effects in PD subjects. There is no doubt that these exercises can help to prevent atrophy of different tissues and slow the aggravation of functional status in PD subjects. Since the movement difficulty has resulted from BG dysfunction and PD subjects will be less and less reliant on BG to generate movements; it is therefore important that PD subjects learn to perform different functional tasks using movements that are generated by the intact motor areas of the brain.

Another important aspect needs consideration, which is the possibility to foster changes in the brain. Modern brain imaging techniques reveal that human brain is endowed with plastic changes, which include experience-dependent change and functional reorganisation. The use of movement strategies to minimise different task difficulty at home may facilitate those changes in the intact neural circuits of the brain in PD subjects. The advantages of adapting home based movement strategies are that they do not only help PD subjects to counteract the underlying factors that are responsible the producing functional disability but also the repeated use of those tasks during daily life activities may facilitate changes in the intact neural circuits. Holden et al (2006), Morris et al (1998), Carr and Shepherd (2004) have affirmed that motor learning literatures show that skills are learned most effectively when they are practiced repeatedly in relation to meaningful goals. Moreover research on neural adaptation has demonstrated that goal directed and learning-based training can contribute to enhanced function in people with neurodegenerative condition (Tillerson et al 2002). It is clear that adapting the movement strategies during three principal tasks at home can be a good opportunity for many PD subjects to repeat them during different activities of daily living; moreover they are part of meaningful goal directed activities. In addition these movement strategies bypass the involvement of BG and use intact areas of the brain. It is therefore assumed that those intact areas may in long-term be reorganised and can compensate the functional losses resulted from BG dysfunction. However PD is a degenerative condition and the possibility to facilitate neural change and to maintain functional autonomy in people with this disease is unknown. Moreover an intact cognitive function plays an important role in facilitating neural change, whereas many PD subject may have wide range of cognitive impairment and it is not clear how much neural changes can be facilitate to achieve a long-term functional improvement. Therefore a clinical research can help to identify whether PD subjects can learn an alternative movement strategy to change their functional status.

II

A Brief Anatomy Physiology of Basal Ganglia and Some Associated Motor Areas

Parkinson's disease is characterised by cell loss and gliosis in a paired brain stem nucleus called the substantia nigra (Jellinger 1986, Forno1996). Due to a progressive loss of substantia nigra neurons that produce dopamine, imbalances occur in the basal ganglia (Greenfield and Bosanquet 1953), and people began to experience difficulties with motor skills, cognition, and automatic function (Hughes et al 1993). It is now widely accepted that through their interaction with the cerebral cortex the basal ganglia also contribute to variety of behaviour and cognitive functions other than voluntary movements (Kandel et al 2000). Therefore it is clear that different PD symptoms become apparent due to the imbalance of dopamine in the basal ganglia of the brain. It is clear that neurotransmitter impairment within the BG and their connection is responsible for the PD symptoms, and that the symptoms include motor as well as cognitive impairment. It is an essential aspect to understand the function of each area of basal ganglia; and the areas that are affected as well the areas remain unaffected can one establish the optimal routes for the stimulation in order to foster changes ('experience-dependent change' Gould et al 1999, and 'functional reorganisation' Nudo et al 2001) in the intact neural circuits. Robertson (1999) suggests that neuroscience can make it significant contribution toward the development of scientific basis for the practice of brain rehabilitation through elucidating the brain's functional architecture. The following discussion reviews briefly the different cells of basal ganglia, their connections as well as their functions. Moreover the supplementary motor area, premotor area, and primary motor area of the cerebral cortex have functions akin to basal ganglia function and it may be possible that the function of those areas may be reorganised to compensate functional losses resulted from basal ganglia degeneration.

II 1. The nuclei of basal ganglia:

A cluster of cell bodies within deeper level of the brain along with their connections is responsible for the motor and non-motor activities; and those neurons together are identified as basal ganglia. The four principal nuclei of basal ganglia include (1) the striatum (caudate nucleus, putamen); (2) the globus pallidus; (3) the substantia nigra; and (4) the sub thalamic nucleus. According to Meara and Bhowmic (2000) the substenti nigra is a pigmented dopamine rich nucleus that forms part of closely related deep-seated subcortical brain brain nuclei, collectively called the basal ganglia. The substantia nigra consists of a densely cellular pars compacta, and a less cellular pars reticulata, again pars reticulate forms a major output nucleus of the basal ganglia projecting to specific thalamic nuclei and receiving afferent inputs from the straitum and sbthalamic nucleus (Meara and Koller 2000). In PD the absence pigmented substentia nigra cells are observed. Kandel et al (2000) suggests that putamen is an important site for integration of movement related to sensory feedback information.

II2. Connections of basal ganglia:

The functional anatomy of the basal ganglia may be defined in terms of several functional loops which comprises of different feed-forward and feedback pathway between basal ganglia and themselves and basal ganglia and other cortical areas (Alexader et al 1986). The basal ganglia themselves and in association with other areas of cerebral cortex through different connection, are responsible for wide range motor and non motor functions.

II 2a Connection of basal ganglia within themselves:

The nerve fibres from the substantia nigra terminate at the level of neostraitum (putamen and caudate nucleus) and secret dopamine at their nerve endings and on the other hand nerve fibres from the neostraitum terminate at the level of substantia nigra and these fibres secret an inhibitory neurotransmitter, called GABA, at their nerve endings (Guyton 1981). Therefore this connection loop within the basal ganglia is responsible for the certain degree of inhibition of muscle activity or the tonicity of muscles.

II2b. Connection of basal ganglia and other areas of brain:

The motor sings of PD appear to the result from a failure of the motor loop that that links the sensoriomotor cortex, putamen, globus pallidus, substantia nigra, pars reticula, thalamus and the supplementary motor areas in the cortex. These nuclei receive their primary input from cerebral cortex and send their output to the brain stem and, via the thalamus, back to the prefrontal, premotor, and motor cortices (Kandel et al 2000). The authors further suggest that the basal ganglia have extensive and highly organised connections with virtually the entire cerebral cortex, as well as the hippocampus and amygdala whereas the basal ganglia have relatively few connections to the brain stem and no direct connection at all to the spinal cord. Moreover the basal ganglia may be viewed as then principal subcortical components of a family of circuit linking the thalamus and cerebral cortex. The basic output from the thalamus is excitatory to the cortex, though this can be altered by the inputs from the output nuclei of the basal ganglia, which causes tonic inhibition of the thalamus. The following are five connection loop of basal ganglia and other areas of the brain and their specific function:

1. The skeletomotor circuit: it originates in the cerebral cortex in precentral motor fields (the premotor cortex and supplementary motor area, and the motor cortex) and project largely to the putamen and ends back to the precentral motor fields; this circuits has subcircuits centred on different

precentral motor fields, with separate somatotopic pathways for control of leg, arm, and orofacial movements (Kandel et al 2000). Afifi (1993) suggests that disruption of this circuit may result pure motor deficit of the leg arm and orofacial movements.

2. The occulomotor circuit begins and ends in the frontal and supplementary eye fields. The frontal eye fields and several other cortical areas project to the body of caudate and then they end up at the frontal eye field via the thalamus; and this circuit is involved in the control of saccadic eye movements (Kandel et al 1991); similarly according to Afifi (1993) the disruption of this circuit results pure motor deficit. However Fuster (1980) suggests that this circuit is involved in the distribution of visual and spatial attention.
3. The prefrontal circuit begins in the dorsolateral prefrontal and lateral orbito frontal cortex and several other areas of association cortex project to the dorsolateral head of the caudate nucleus and projects back to the dorsolateral prefrontal cortex via the thalamus Kandel et al (1991). They further affirm that that this circuit is probably involved in aspect of memory concerned with orientation and executive function; and the damage to the dorsolateral prefrontal cortex or sub-cortical portions is associated with variety of behavioural abnormalities related to these cognitive functions.
4. Lateral orbitofrontal circuit; this circuit originates and ends up in the lateral orbitofrontal cortex, via the ventromedial caudate nucleus. The lateral orbitofrontal circuit might be involved in switches in behavioural set (Fuster 1980). According to Kandel et al (2000) damage to this area is associated with irritability, emotional liability, failure to response to social cues, and lack of empathy.
5. Limbic circuit begins and ends in the anterior cingulated area and medial orbito frontal cortex. According to Afifi (1993) disruption of this circuit may result in emotional deficit. Damage to this region bilaterally can cause akinetic mutism, a condition characterised by profound impairment of movement initiation.

III

Function of Basal Ganglia

Neurons of basal ganglia along with their connections regulate a wide range of motor, cognitive, and behaviour functions. Three distinct characteristics of basal ganglia enable them perform to these functions. These characteristics include, - secretion of neurotransmitter, - maintain a wide range of connection with the other parts of the brain, - and finally they function as a storing and retrieving structure of learned motor activities.

II3a. Secretion of neurotransmitter:

Hornykiewicz (1966) found that in patients with Parkinson's disease the content of dopamine, norepinephrine, and serotonin was low and of these three biogenic amines, dopamine was most drastically low. In addition to the dopaminergic projection to the neostriatum, there are also dopaminergic projections to parts of the limbic system and the frontal neocortex (Kandel et al 1991), and those areas have important role in the initiation of movements and regulation of some specific cognitive functions. Therefore the lack of dopamine on those parts of the brain is responsible for the PD symptoms. Kandel et al (1991) further affirms that the akinesia seen in patients with PD may be due partly to dopamine depletion in the limbic system, especially in the nucleus accumbens. However recent evidence suggests that the loss of striatal dopamine account for most of the symptoms, in PD there are also losses of noradrenergic neurons in the locus ceruleus and serotonergic neurons in the raphe nuclei (Kandel et al 1991). It is clear that that there PD is not only degeneration of the dopamine producing neurons but also there can be degeneration of neurons in the other areas of BG. Presumably PD starts with the degeneration dopamine producing neurons(substantia nigra) and progressively the degenerative process may extends to the other areas of the brain. Moreover some of the specific cognitive deficits of the disease may also be due to loss of dopamine from the nerve endings in the cortex (Kandel 1991). Therefore it is evident that not only muscle rigidity but also other functions like initiation of movements, and cognitive functions may also be affected due to the lack of dopamine.

II3b. Connection with different areas of the brain:

The basal ganglia are connected to and from the different areas of the brain, and these circuits form valuable anatomic and physiologic framework. They are responsible not only for diverse motor activities but also for wide range of cognitive and behavioural functions. Moreover these circuits are largely segregated structurally and functionally (Kandel et al 2000), which may explain the dissimilarity of symptoms between individual PD subjects.

II3C. Function of basal ganglia as storing and retrieving structure of motor activities:

In the early stages of skill acquisition, frontal cortical regions are used to control movements using attentional processes (Seitz 1992, Jueptner et al 1997); with practice, control is relegated to the basal ganglia,(Holden et al 2006, Galletly and Brauer 2005, Jueptner et al 1997), which then function as storing and retrieving structure of learned motor skills. In other word the basal ganglia are responsible for the generation of previously learned movements as well as modulating and organising precisely shaped movements. The motor skills are stored in BG, which can be retrieved without involving cortical region, or without using attentional process, and which in turn enable one to perform different functional tasks quickly, easily, and spontaneously. Marsden (1982) affirms that the basal ganglia are responsible for the automatic execution of learned motor plan. Luria (1973) suggests that selective perceiving and responding of different functional tasks are the function of BG. Therefore when the basal ganglia are dysfunctional, these learned movements are no longer available for automatic execution, leading to a disruption of kinematic organisation of motor activities (Kinematic motor organisation is the interrelated and interdependent motor activities, which constitute the essential organisational structure for performing functional tasks). Moreover dopamine as neurotransmitter plays most vital role for the proper function of basal ganglia neurons. It may be concluded that dopamine plays most important role for the proper functioning of basal ganglia, and lack of dopamine is responsible for the production of PD symptoms.

II 4 The role of neurotransmitter for the proper functioning of the basal ganglia and their connection and some underlying factors responsible for the Parkinson disease symptoms:

The dopamine constitutes an essential neurotransmitter for the proper functioning of the basal ganglia neurons and their connections. The brains of patients with Parkinson disease have loss of nerve cells and depigmentation of substantia nigra, and the severity of change in the substantia nigra parallels the reduction of dopamine in the in the straitum (Kandel et al 1991). Experiments on animals show that the Parkinsonian symptoms are produced more easily by altering transmitter systems, which causes an abnormal output from the basal ganglia, than by the lesion in basal ganglia, which eliminate the output; and therefore, it is likely that the underlying pathology of disorder basal ganglia in human is a disruption of transmitter metabolism (Kandel et al 1991). Meara and Koller (2000) affirm that loss of dopaminergic modulation in the straitum causes profound disturbances of voluntary motor control leading to akinesia, tremour and rigidity.

The underlying factor responsible for the parkinsonian symptoms is the paucity of dopamine in the BG. Dopamine has two important functions, - it neutralises acetylcholine, and works as an essential neurotransmitter for the functioning of the basal ganglia and their connections with the other parts of the brain. Aetylcholine has stimulating effect on the motor neurons of the brain, therefore in the absence of dopamine result in excess of acetylcholine in the brain, which in turn provokes contraction of antagonist and agonist muscles producing muscle rigidity. The neurotransmitter lack is responsible for the dysfunction of BG, which inturn responsible for the breakdown of the kinematic organisation of motor activities. In other words the organised motor program are no longer available for execution. The akinesia seen in patients with Parkinson's disease may be due to dopamine depletion in the limbic system, and some of the specific cognitive deficits in the disease may also be due to loss dopamine from nerve endings in the cortex (Kandel et al 1991).

Greenfield and Bosanquet (1953) state that due to a progressive loss of substantia nigra neurons that produce dopamine, neurotransmitter imbalances occur in the basal ganglia. Once around 80% of the neurons have been lost, PD symptoms become evident and people begin to experience difficulties with motor skills, cognition, and automatic function (Hughes et al 1993). Moreover Kandel et al (1991) suggests in Parkinson's disease as many as 90% of the dopaminergic neurons degenerate. The administration of dopamine helps to enhance the function of the BG and minimise the PD symptoms. However Kandel et al (1991) state that L-DOPA therapy has been hailed as the most significant advance in the treatment of Parkinson's disease, it has not been the panacea hoped for when it was first introduced; at that time it was hoped that L-DOPA might not only ameliorate the symptoms of Parkinson's disease, but also reverse some of the degenerative changes seen in the substantia nigra. This does not happen; L-DOPA only controls some of the symptoms; it does not alter the course of the disease. In addition many patients become refractory or suffer side effects after treatment with L-DOPA for several years (Kandel et al 1991). It is therefore essential to identify the strategies, which may enable PD subjects to reduce the dependency on high dose of L-DOPA. How L-DOPA ameliorates the symptoms of

PD is still unclear (Kandel et al 1991). The authors further state that presumably the L-dopa is taken up and converted into dopamine by the remaining dopaminergic nerve cells; the few healthy dopamiergic neurons and those that have partially degenerated may be able to compensate by carrying out the entire function of the nigrostraital system. Moreover heavy external admistration of dopamine may be responsible for the functional deprivation of the remaining healthy and partially degenerated nigrostraital system, enhancing their degenerative process. There remains paucity of evidence suggesting the aggravation of atrophy and degenerative process of partially healthy remaining dopaminergic system.

Disruption of neurotransmission function, liked to depletion dopamine within the BG and their connection produces PD symptoms. Although the administration of oral dopamine minimise the symptoms in the initial stage of the disease process, its long-term effect is minimum. In contrast prolong high dose of dopamine may enhance the atrophy and degeneration the remaining healthy and partially degenerated nigrostraital system. of

II4. Role of different motor areas in generating movements:

Imbalance of dopamine, which is a neurotransmitter within the BG is responsible for production of Parkinson symptoms. This neurotransmitter is responsible for the proper functioning of different connections within the BG and the connections between BG and the other motor areas of the brain. Kendal et al (2000) suggest that motor actions of the basal ganglia are mediated in large part through the supplementary, premotor and motor cortices via the pyramidal system. Moreover Luria (1973) suggests that the kinetic organisation of movements depends on the combined activity of basal ganglia and the premotor area. The kinetic organisation of movement may be disrupted due to the lack of dopamine within BG. Therefore dopamine lack within the BG not only impaired BG function but also the circuits that constitute by the BG, premotor, supplementary motor, pyramidal system can be disrupted. However the other motor areas remain unaffected at least at the initial stage of the disease process in PD subjects. It is therefore worthwhile to investigate if the functioning of those areas can be upheld independent of BG's involvement. The following discussion reviews the functions of theses motor areas.

The supplementary motor area is possibly involved in the preparation and execution of complex voluntary movements, especially if these movements are learned, and thus be responsible for the internal cuing and guidance of acquired skilled motor acts of the limbs (Roland et al 1980, Chen et al 1995, Thalar et al 1995). Therefore supplementary motor area plays an important role in the initiation of movements, and a functional reorganisation in the supplementary motor area may help PD subject to overcome this initiation difficulty.

However supplementary motor area is probably activated by the stimulation from basal ganglia. Alexander and Crutcher (1990) affirm that the neural projections from the internal segment of globus pallidus of basal ganglia to the supplementary motor area and primary motor cortex secrets neurotransmitters and responsible for the preparation of movements and termination of movements. Therefore it is important to identify the possibility to activate supplementary motor area by bypassing the involvement of basal ganglia.

Moreover premotor area is probably involved in coupling environmental cues to motor acts and may be responsible to external stimuli (Chen et al 1995). Endogenous movements (previously learned movements) are mainly mediated by supplementary motor area activity, while initiation of externally referenced movements is the role of pre-motor cortex neurones.

Furthermore Weissenborn (1995) suggests that supplementary motor area and premotor areas are activated prior to voluntary movement and the impairment of supplementary motor area appears to reflect the activity of impaired basal ganglia. These two areas are responsible for generation of many spontaneous muscle activities. The supplementary motor area is critical regulating the increase in neural activity that needs to occur before a movement is executed; moreover they ensure that movement is terminated in appropriate time (Brochie et al 1991; Cunnington et al 1995). In the case of damage to the BG/SMA pathways PD subjects rely heavily on intact sensory/PMA pathways to initiate movements (Georgiou et al 1993) Moreover Primary motor cortex controls muscle force and the direction of movement (Liston and Tallis 2000). Primary motor cortex along with premotor area may generate movement in response to external sensory stimuli like visual, auditory and proprioceptive information. Marseden (1989) suggests that in the case of damaged BG/SMA pathways, these pathways could be bypassed by sensory information from the environment feeds directly into PMA through visual, auditory and proprioceptive pathways and the premotor area subsequently activate the primary motor cortex. The finding of Papa et al (1991) indicates that not only visual cues but also auditory and somato-sensory afferents can trigger the primary motor cortex without supplementary motor area activation. Therefore it may be assumed that the kinetic organisation of movements can be facilitated by external sensory stimulation, and by bypassing BG involvement.

Conclusion: It can be concluded that the basal ganglia are the clusters of neurons deep in the brain structure. They have three distinct functions, which are – secretion of neurotransmitter, dopamine; - assure connection with the other areas of the other areas of the brain and finally; - they function as storing and retrieving structure of learned motor activities. Therefore retrieving difficulty of learned movement can cause difficulty to perform functional tasks. The neurons of BG have extensive connection with different part of cerebral cortex and hypothalamus, which is the reason that the basal ganglia not only regulate motor activities but also responsible for the cognitive aspect of motor control. Moreover these connections are functionally and structurally segregated, which may explain that different Parkinson subjects have different symptoms. The supplementary motor area plays an important role in the initiation and termination of movements. Furthermore the symptoms of impaired of supplementary motor area appears to reflect the activity of impaired basal ganglia. It may be assumed that a functional reorganisation of these areas may compensate the functional loss of basal ganglia.

IV

Diagnosis of Parkinson's Disease

Parkinson's disease is characterised by three principal symptoms, which are akinesia of movements, rigidity of muscles and tremor at rest. To identify patients with Parkinsonism correctly it is important to be able to recognise correctly the cardinal clinical features of PD, namely akinesia, lead pipe rigidity, rest tremor, and postural instability (Rodnitzky 2000).

According to Rodnitzky (2000) akinsia is reduction of spontaneous and automatic motor activity, slow movements, and difficulty with sequential and concurrent motor acts, abnormal early fatigability and reduction in amplitude of movements. A lack of facial expression attended by reduced blink rate is one of the most apparent manifestations of akinesia (Rodnitzky 2000). The clinical signs of akinesia are so striking that their presence alone has been considered by some to be sufficient to establish a diagnosis of PD (Quinn 1995). Akinesia or slowness of movement results from a combination of movement dysfunctions, such as difficulty to initiate and execute movements, difficulty to perform large amplitude movements, difficulty to perform concurrent movements, absence of automatic and spontaneous movements. Different factors of akinesia are responsible for the difficulty to get in and out of a chair, difficulty to get in and out of a bed, difficulty to walk in a confined space. Therefore rigidity of muscles and resting tremor along with difficulty to perform different tasks like getting in and out of the bed, getting in and out of a chair and walking in a confined space are the symptoms of Parkinson's disease. Rodnitzky (2000) affirms that akinesi produces diminished arm swing on one or both sides of the body, difficulty to arising from a chair, a slow, short stepped gait, en block turning, and soft, poorly articulated speech (hypophonia).

Muscle rigidity in PD is characterised by the presence of increased muscle tone in both agonist and antagonist muscle groups. Two types of rigidity usually present in PD, lead pipe rigidity and cog-wheel rigidity (Rodnitzky 2000). Rodnitzky (2000) further describes that lead-pipe rigidity is abnormal resistance which constant throughout the range of movement and is felt when passively stretching muscles around a joint in a relaxed subject, whereas in cog-wheel rigidity a ratchet type of fluctuating resistance felt at the wrist in synchrony with tremor bursts.

Rest tremor is characterised by the presence of a 4-5 Hz oscillation involving the distal portion of the upper limb of 'pill rolling' type (Rodnitzky 2000). However in the condition of 'tremor dominant' PD tremor is an isolated finding and this can easily lead to misdiagnosis with the most common cause of isolated tremor, essential tremor (Rodnitzky 2000). According to Rajput et al (1993) rest tremor, accompanying the most usual postural and kinetic tremor can be a late manifestation of essential tremor in elderly subjects. In PD rest-tremor may be accompanied by postural and kinetic tremors, whereas the head and trunk are usually spared.

Rajput et (1991) found that only 76% of patients with final diagnosis of PD during life had evidence of the disease when examined at autopsy. Hughes et al (1992a) examined 100 brains with final diagnosis of PD could confirm such a diagnosis in only 76% of cases. The diagnosis of the reminder included conditions such as progressive supranuclear palsy (PSP), multiple system atrophy (MSM) and Alzheimer's disease (AD) Therefore Parkinson's Disease society Brain Bank criteria requires the presence of akinesia plus on other clinical singe from among rigidity, rest tremor and postural instability.

V

Early Dementia

Akinesia of movements, muscle rigidity, tremor, and postural instability and falls may be present in other neurological conditions. Dementia is common in PD disease, having been found in as many as 65% patients of by the age of 85years (Mayeux et al 1990). However early dementia in the akinetic-rigid patient should prompt consideration of a variety of other symptoms with parkinsonian features, including dementia with Lewis body (DLB), corticobasal ganglionic degeneration (CBGD), normal pressure hydrocephalus, Creutzfeld-Jacob disease, or Alzheimer's disease (AD) (Rodnitzky 2000). For example in AD dementia is more likely to be associated with abnormality of memory and language and the presence of ansonosia while that of PD is more commonly characterised by impairment of visiospatial and executive functions (Mohr et al 1990, Starkstein et al 1996, Mahieux et al 1998). Similarly hallucination occurring in PD typically appear late in the course of illness and are almost always associated with chronic use of antiparkinsonian drug. However, the hallucination occurring prior to the initiation of such drug or with the first administration of these agents strongly suggests another diagnosis, particularly dementia with Lewy bodies (Rodnitzky 2000).

VI

Fall and Instability in PD

Falling in PD is typically the result of impaired postural reflex, postural hypotension or severe large amplitude dyskinesias, moreover severe freezing with inability to cheque forward propulsion of the upper trunk is another possible cause (Rodnitzky 2000). However conditions like progressive supranuclear palsy (PSP), multiple systemic atrophy (MSA) are conditions which increase the likely hood of falling in people with these conditions. Jankovic et al (1990) describes that the condition among those most likely to present with falling is PSP. Moreover normal pressure hydrocephalus which is characterised by inability to lift the feet from the floor, short shuffling steps, imbalance while walking, difficulty turning, and gait ignition failure (Marsden and Thompson 1997, Graff Rodford and Godersky 1997) may present with frequent fallings.

VII

The Repercussion of Defective Dopamine Metabolism on the Functional Architecture of the Nervous System that Mediates Motor Activities

Human activities are not produced by the action of individual muscle or joint, but they are the result of an organised activity of multiple muscles (kinematic motor organisation). Three distinct motor systems within the functional architecture of the nervous system largely contribute in the structuring of kinematic motor organisation. These systems include, -program control system, which retrieves spontaneously the previously learned muscle activities; - feedback control system, which provides strength and dexterity of individual muscles into the retrieved programmed muscle activities; - and finally the reflex control system, which helps to shape kinematic motor organisation by providing modulated and inhibited reflex muscle activities (detailed description is made in the chapter on Functional architecture of the nervous system that mediates motor activities). As mention earlier that in CVA there is a breakdown of the structure of kinematic motor organisation; in contrast, movement difficulty in PD is the result of a defect in the organisation process while structuring the kinematic motor activities. In particular, a deficit of spontaneous retrieval of program controlled muscle activities. BG neurons are the store house for the previously learned or programmed muscle activities, and with the impaired neurotransmitter metabolism within BG, many PD subjects experience a progressive difficulty of spontaneously retrieving of theses program controlled muscle activities. However, as it is described earlier that despite its spontaneous nature, a series of neural events takes place within the brain while processing, retrieving and executing, in the transforming process of neural activities into a programmed muscle activities. According to Marsden (1984) these events include; - goal identification or stimulus to move; -formulation and organisation of motor program; - initiation of movement and finally; - execution of movement. In PD, one or several of these neural events can be impaired as a result of neurotransmitter metabolism defect at the level of BG. Whereas the spontaneous retrieving of program controlled muscle activities is essential to initiate, adapt, and readapt movements enabling one to perform functional tasks easily and spontaneously. This initiation, adaptation, and re-adaption difficulty in performing functional tasks leads to a progressive decline of activity level and the development of disability in many PD subjects. However when movement analysis is done it unveils that four specific movement dysfunctions are the underlying factors for the initiation, adaptation, and re-adaptation difficulty. These movement dysfunctions are – an impaired background and supporting movements (Khal 1976); -difficulty to initiate and execute movements (Evarts et al 1981, Schimidt 1982); - difficulty to perform large amplitude movements (Beradelli et al 1986, Mak and Col 1991); - difficulty to perform simultaneous movements (Marsden 1984). Moreover certain movement strategies can help PD subjects to minimise the above movement dysfunction and ease the difficulty to perform functional tasks. The following discussion reviews some of the insights of these four major movement dysfunctions, their repercussion on the performance of functional tasks at home and finally the discussion examines the possible movement strategies, which can ease the difficulty task performance within home.

The four movement dysfunctions include:
- Impairment of spontaneous and automatic movements (Khal 1976);
- Difficulty to initiate and execute movements (Evarts et al 1981, Schimidt 1982);

- Difficulty to perform large amplitude movements (Beradelli et al 1986, Mak and Col 1991);
- Difficulty to perform simultaneous movements (Marsden 1984).

The following discussion examines the underlying physiopathology of the four above movement dysfunctions, and the possible strategies for minimizing those difficulties.

Impaired spontaneous and automatic movements:

The basal ganglia are responsible for generating many stereotyped, spontaneous movements during different function tasks (Guyton 1991). As mention earlier that BG neurons are the store house of previously learned activities. These leaned activities are stored as programmed motor activities, and they can be retrieved spontaneously without much voluntary effort. That is activities in the BG launch a series of interconnected and interdependent muscle activities to achieve a desired functional task. According to Khal (1976) these muscle actions are neither voluntary nor conscious (more detail discussion is made in the chapter on program control system of the brain). In the absence of these automatic and spontaneous movements, the voluntary movements are left alone to function and consequently voluntary movements act with a different rhythm and the overall tasks are much more fatigable (Bleton 1985). For example, during walking automatic dissociation of pelvic and pectoral girdles, dorsiflexion of the ankle, and erection of the vertebral column and even swinging of the arms constitute the involuntary and background movement, which helps to perform walking smoothly in a spontaneous manner. In the absence of these movements the PD subjects walk with flexion of vertebral column, there is absence of dissociation of pelvic and pectoral girdles, and in the absence of automatic dorsiflexion of the ankle the whole foot arrives on the ground (normal walking consists of heel strike, mid stance and push off by the toes). Another example is standing from the sitting position, where one automatically pulls both feet backwards, leans forward in order to facilitate standing. Whereas in case of people with PD the feet remain in front of the line of gravity of the body, the head stays behind the line of gravity because of absence of spontaneous and automatic flexion of the trunk and the knees before getting out of the chair. Probably basal ganglia along with glutometergic of pedunculo pontine neurones (PPN) are responsible for the generation of the automatic, background movements. Pahapill and Lazano (2000) suggest that PPN is thought to be important regulator of basal ganglia and spinal cord and these neurons thought to be involved in the modulation of gait and other stereotyped movements and PD subjects have significant loss of PPN. This movement difficulty may be minimised to a certain extent if PD subjects can learn to use voluntary movements to replace involuntary, background movements.

Difficulty to initiate and execute movements:

The difficulty to perform movements in PD may be due to delay in the initiation (reaction time) and execution of movements (movement time). Reaction time (RT) is the measure of the time elapsed from the presentation of stimulus to the beginning of a response to stimulus, whereas movement time is the time taken in the execution once it is initiated (Schimidt 1982). Evert et al (1981) have reported the evaluation of RT using a visual signal of pronation-supination of the forearm. A higher degree of variability both between subjects and within subjects at different times of the day was detected. These result appear to suggest that the time take to initiate a movement (reaction time) and the time take to execute a movement (movement time) are prolonged in people with PD. Overall, movement time was reported to be more consistently and profoundly affected than reaction time. Sheridan et al (1987) studied choice reaction time by adding different degrees of accuracy constrain to the responses required. The increase of in response complexity may have the difficulty of the motor programming process. The subjects were instructed to make movements to a target, and simple and choice reaction times were measured. The result of this investigation showed that pre-motor reaction time was significantly longer in people with PD than for age-matched controls in the simple reaction time condition (pre-motor reaction time is defied the interval between the onset of the stimulus and the first sign of heightened EMG activity) (Weiss 1965). These experiments show that people with PD have deficits in the initiation and execution of movement and the difficulty can aggravate where the movement requires different degree of accuracy. However when a movement requires different degree of accuracy using attention can minimise the deficit of initiation and execution. Therefore not only initiation and execution defect are responsible for the slowness of movements but also a defective attention function is responsible for the slowness of movements. According to Marsden (1989) the slowness of movement is caused by the disorder of timing mechanism of movement that may be due to inability to hold or deliver motor programs with normal speed. It seems the previously stored, programmed activities from the BG fail to transform in to muscle action due to deficit of neurotransmission between BG and cortical motor areas. It is clear that several underlying factors seem to be responsible for the difficulty to initiate and execute movement PD subjects, which include:

- An breakdown of connection between BG to motor cortical areas;
- An impaired of neurotransmitter metabolism within basal ganglia neurons;
- An attention dysfunction;

Difficulty to initiate movement due to breakdown of connection between basal ganglia and cortical motor area:

A breakdown in the connection of basal ganglia and the cortical motor areas seems to be responsible for the delay in the initiation and execution of movements. In fact there may not a real break down of connection, rather a breakdown of transmission of action potential from the BG to the cortical motor areas. According to Mak and Col (1991) in PD the delay in the response initiation may be due to impairment in the organisation or translation of motor programs in to muscle actions. Therefore they suggest that the subjects with PD appear to have no difficulty in selection and formulation of motor programme there is a breakdown in the connection between BG and cortical motor areas. There may be no impairment in the selection and construction of motor program, the output of the motor program may be inaccurate because of faulty integration with in the cortical centres (Mak and Col 1991). That is, there appear to be breakdown of the link between perceptual appreciation of what is needed and delivery of appropriate instructions to the motor cortex, which may due to the interruption within the connection between the basal ganglia and the motor cortex (Mak and Col 1991). Earlier Beradelli et al (1986) also affirmed that it is the command sent to the cortex, which appears to be incorrect. That is, there is no impairment in the selection and construction level, but the information does not reach up to the motor cortex, which in turn fails to produce appropriate movements required to meet the specific demands of the environment or the desired goal of the performer. This interruption is caused by lack of neurotransmitter, eventually hindering the propagation of action potential from the BG to motor cortical areas. It can therefore be concluded that the breakdown of transmission of action potential between BG and cortical motor areas is responsible for the faulty organisation or translation of motor programs in to appropriate muscle action; that the breakdown can create a deficit in the perceptual appreciation of what is needed and delivery of appropriate instructions to the motor cortex. These impairments in turn are responsible for delay in initiation and execution of movements.

Difficulty to initiate movement due to lack of dopamine within the basal ganglia neurons:

Another theory suggests that lack of dopamine within the BG can be responsible for the delayed initiation of movements. When body performs a muscle activity, action potentials appear in the basal ganglia before they appear in the cortical motor areas, and it is likely that the basal ganglia themselves are set into activity not by the signal from the motor cortex but instead by signals directly from sensory and sensory association portion of the cortex; or from thalamus and brain stem (Guyton 1981). Thus, there is much belief that the basal ganglia neurons play an essential role in the initiation of most if not all the motor activities of the body (Guyton 1981). Most probably the four neural events within the BG, which are - goal identification or stimulus to move; -formulation and organisation of motor program; - initiation of movement and; - execution of movement, do not take place due to lack of dopamine. As a result, the stored motor programmes may either be difficult to be retrieved or they may simply are not be available for automatic execution. Sheridan (1987) suggests that the motor program is not lost entirely; aspect of it may need to be recomputed. The author further reports that in a simple reaction time situation, those with PD are likely to be slower to initiate movement, and more variable in the time taken to initiate the movement than age matched normal controls. However it is observed a wide range of variability in the initiation of movements and the ability to adapt and readapt in the environment during different tasks among the PD subjects. Consequently the lack of dopamine within BG provokes difficulty to perform learned motor skills like walking, getting in and out of the bed, getting in and out of a chair. Morris (2000) affirms that dopamine apparently plays a role in allowing people to execute well-learned skilled movements smoothly and quickly. Therefore the pre-programmed motor activities may become difficult to be retrieved because of lack of dopamine within BG. This eventually can contribute to the slowness to initiate and execute movements.

The role of attention in initiation and execution of movements:

Part of basal ganglia neurons and their connections also contribute in regulating attention function, and therefore the lack of dopamine may engender an impair attention function. Goodrich et al (1989) studied the ability to use advance information for controlling movement in PD subjects. They contrasted the simple and the choice reaction time, in medicated PD subjects with mild and moderate affection with that of healthy controls. The principal finding converge on the notion that the deficit in simple reaction time was due to impairment of an attention demanding process which facilitates reaction time performance when required response was known in advance. Moreover large differences exist between PD subjects and controls in task requiring movement preparation and movement execution (Van Zomeren and Brouwer 1994). It is described in the chapter on program control system that attention function is activated while performing complicated tasks. For example walking in an unknown or uneven terrain, the role of selective attention plays crucial role in retrieving and structuring the interrelated and interdependent muscle activities. In contrast many PD subjects with the difficulty to spontaneous initiation and execution of learned movements, they may rely on attention function to overcome the task difficulty; however PD subjects with impaired attention function may be unable to minimise their task difficulty. Morris (2000) affirms that PD subjects with intact attention function are able to minimise their movement difficulties by focusing attention on the crucial aspect of the movement. Therefore people with impair attention will have difficulty to initiate and execute movement and they will experience extra difficulty to adapt movements in a difficult terrain or in an unknown environment. In addition the experience dependent-dependent plastic reorganisation depends on attention being paid by the recipient to the stimulation responsible for such changes (Recanzone et al 1993: [Recanzone, G.H. Schreiner, C.E. and Merzenich, M.M. (1993) plasticity in the frequency representation of primary auditory cortex, Journal of Neuroscience, 13, P87-103]. Therefore an impaired attention function not only results in difficulty to initiate and execute movements, but also plastic changes in the intact neural circuits of the brain will be hindered. Thus PD subjects with impaired attention are observed that their level of functional decline is accelerated. Some PD subjects with attention dysfunction can minimise initiation and execution difficulty to a certain extent by using visual and verbal stimulation, probably these sensory stimulations help to compensate impaired attention function.

Neurotransmitter metabolism defect at the level of connection between BG and cortical motor areas is responsible for the failure to transformation motor program into motor action, provoking difficulty to initiate organised activity of the task. Moreover BG themselves fail to be activated to generate programmed activities, due to lack of neurotransmitter within them. Attention function also plays important role in the initiation and execution of movements therefore PD subjects with impaired attention can experience difficulty to adapt with their movement difficulty and their decline is of accelerated because they are unable to foster experience d-dependent change in the intact neural circuit.

Difficulty to perform large amplitude movements:

Several studies have demonstrated the evidence of slowness of movements with larger amplitude in subjects with PD. For example according to Beradelli et al (1986) the delay in the first phase ballistic movement may have been due to inappropriate scaling of the agonist burst to suit movement amplitude. According to Mak and Cole (1991) the movement of greater amplitude and precision would take a longer time to execute because of the difficulty to processing the information during the movement. In normal individuals the reaction time (reaction time is the measure of the time elapsed from the presentation of stimulus to the beginning of a response to stimulus) become longer with increased movement distance and degree of terminal accuracy (Glencross 1977 and Klapp 1975), which they compensate either by decreasing average velocity (Flankenberg and Newell 1980) or by increasing the number of response components (Fischman 1984). However PD subjects with defective BG function can neither increase the number of response component, nor they can adapt the velocity of movement; instead they often reduce the amplitude of movement.

Moreover larger the amplitude of movement more it requires the number of interdependent and interrelated components of motor activities. The inability to generate sufficient number of interrelated and interdependent muscle actions due to impaired neurotransmitter metabolism within BG, PD subjects often tend to use voluntary effort to execute the entire movement, that is they use the intact feedback control motor activities. However the feedback control muscle activities are not the part of interrelated and interdependent structure of programmed motor activities. In contrast they provide the strength and dexterity in to the pre-programmed movement structure; they are also designed to provide the added parameter in generalised motor program to specify the details of the movements. Therefore use of feedback control movement can have an interfering effect on large amplitude movement and can produce 'hastening'. Hömberg (1993) explains that movement with large amplitude PD subjects cannot cover the entire frequency range of rhythmic movements, when the frequency of tapping is increased, for example, patients with PD reach a certain point where they can no longer follow the target frequency but instead jump into a much higher frequency and this phenomenon is usually called "hastening." Therefore in PD subjects the difficulty to execute of large amplitude of movements results from an inappropriate scaling of agonist-antagonist burst to suit movement amplitude; moreover PD subjects cannot adapt by increasing response component or reducing velocity of movement in case of a large amplitude movements; and finally the larger the amplitude of movement more the interrelated and interdependent motor components are involved, and the defective BG have difficulty in generating several components of superimposed motor activities.

Difficulty to perform complicated and simultaneous movements:

The analyses of sequential and simultaneous movement in PD subjects reveal that motor plans and programs are impaired (Hömberg 1993). "It has been repeatedly demonstrated that impaired in performance of simultaneous and sequential movements beyond and above the impairment shown in performing isolated movements" (Goldenberg et al 1990 P 139). However the reasons for the impairment of more complex movements in PD are often equivocal. It may be that when added together the impairment in execution of each simple movement in complex task exaggerates the deficit in the total task (Mak and col 1991); or it may be a deficit in information processing and organisation of motor plan, which results in greater difficulty in the performance of complex task (Marsden 1984). Holden et al (2006) and Rauch (1997) state that the role of the caudate in processing multiple sensory stimuli and motor skill learning is disrupted in PD. Moreover according to Mak and col (1991) the extra-slowness in the execution of complicated concurrent movement appear to be result of deficits in switching of one programme to another with in a motor plan in sequential movements, or in superimposition of motor programs to form a motor plan in simultaneous movements. Kinematic analysis of the basic functional tasks like getting in and out of a bed, getting in and out of and chair reveal that each task has its own organisational structure, and components of movements are interrelated and dependent on each other. In the process of retrieving programmed activities the BG play important role in prioritising one muscle action, while suppress others among the different interrelated and interdependent muscle activities, in order to produce a successful functional task. However tasks like walking and turning or turning to get in and out of a room involve the mediation of multiple programs, and can be considered as multiple program tasks. In a multiple program task BG neuron not only mediate in selecting and prioritising one muscle action and suppress others, but also they are involved in prioritising one programme and suppressing others among several programs. In normal situation, as the multiple programmes become complicate the BG use selective attention to facilitate the process of selecting and prioritising program. Denny-Brown and Yanagisawa (1976) suggest that an important role of basal ganglia is that they regulate selective attention, which functions as "clearinghouse" that accumulates samples of ongoing cortical activity and, on a competitive basis, can facilitate any one and suppress the others. That is, attention function mediates in prioritising one action and suppresses others within multiple interrelated and interdependent muscle activities in order to accomplish a successful functional task. A simple task or a single programmed task is retrieved spontaneously without the involvement of attention function; however a complicated task or a multi-programmed task, the selective attention gets involved in prioritising and selecting process in spontaneous performance of task. A routine task the BG neurons function independently without involving selective attention in retrieving the organised motor activities. However in a complex task walking new environment, or walking and turning, that is a multiple programmed task, the attention function gets involved as a 'clearinghouse' effectively prioritising and selecting muscle action. Moreover Flowers and Robertson (1985) suggest Parkinson subjects might have difficulty in suppressing the previously irrelevant response and focusing attention on a new response. Whereas according to Mak and Col (1991) there appear to have deficit in switching attention from one motor program to another in the sequential task. Therefore it can be assumed that PD subjects may be able to minimise task difficulty by focusing attention to the main aspect of task. Cunning (2005) has demonstrated that walking performance was improved when people with PD attended to walking, as opposed to attending concurrent tasks. In this study walking performance in people with PD was temporarily improved by directing attention towards a more internal focus (that is focusing on their own movements of maintaining big steps) compared to directing attention towards a more external focus. Another strategy might be to disintegrate multiple program tasks into several single program tasks. Therefore PD subjects with intact selective attention may be able to minimise difficulty of performing complicated simultaneous tasks by using attention function.

It can be concluded that extra slowness is observed while performing simultaneous concurrent movements and in PD subjects. This slowness is because complex tasks consist of several simple tasks, therefore several simple task-difficulties exaggerate the total task difficulty. The task difficulty also link to a deficit of BG in switching one motor program to another in the organisation of motor plan. And finally the task difficulty is due to an impaired selective attention, given that the selective attention plays important role in selecting and prioritising task among a complex task.

Conclusion: Each functional task has its own organisation structure, which consists of a series of interrelated and interdependent muscle activities. These organisational structures are stored in the BG as programmed activity and the whole program can be retrieved to attain a functional objective or to meet specific demand of the environment. Neurotransmitter metabolism deficit within BG results in a difficulty to retrieve these programmed activities, rendering it difficult to perform different functional tasks. Difficulty to retrieve spontaneously the pre-programmed motor activities, many PD subjects become more dependent of voluntary or feedback controlled activities in performing tasks. Therefore they do not only function differently, but also experience difficulty to perform functional tasks. The task difficulty in turn is responsible for the reduced activity level and the development of disability in many PD subjects. However movement analysis in PD subjects unveils, that the defective retrieval of programmed activities results in four distinct movement dysfunctions which include a difficulty to perform spontaneous movements; the difficulty to initiate and execute movements; the difficulty to perform large amplitude movements; finally an extra difficulty to perform simultaneous and complicated movements. Moreover some of the above movement dysfunctions can be minimised, and many

PD subjects can reduce their functional difficulty up to a certain extent. For example the difficulty initiate and execute movements can be minimise to a certain extent when PD subjects learn use sensory and cognitive strategies; the difficulty to perform complicated and concurrent tasks can be minimised by disintegrating them in to several simple tasks; or overcome the difficulty to perform large amplitude movements PD subjects learn to identify the optimal cuing frequency to avoid miscalling The next chapter examines some of the movement strategies that enable PD subjects to minimise the underlying movement difficulties will be examined in detailed.

Movement strategies to minimise the four distinct movement difficulties in PD subjects:

The discussion in the previous chapter has highlighted that there exist four distinct movement dysfunctions. In this chapter the discussion will include some of the movement strategies that can minimise those difficulties. Morris (2000) suggests that the physical therapy intervention in people with PD is based on the assumption that the normal movement can be generated by teaching patients strategy to bypass the basal ganglia pathology. Because cortical regions remain unaffected by the disease in the early stages, the person appears to be able to use "online" frontal-lobe cognitive strategies to compensate for BG insufficiency. Furthermore one striking features in PD is that the ability to move is not lost; rather there is an activation problem (Iansek et al 1995, Martin 1967). Moreover in people who are cognitively intact, simply focusing on attention on the critical aspect of movement that needs to be controlled can be sufficient to activate movements with near-normal speed and size (Morris et al 1996, Behrman et al, Morris et al 1998) 37,40,42 Morris (2000).Therefore it may be assumed that people with intact cognitive function may be able to change their functional status by integrating movement strategies like conscious voluntary effort, attention function, and external sensory cues, during different functional tasks. It can also be assumed that in PD, where basal ganglia function is defective, practice and repetitive use of voluntary effort, attention strategy, and external sensory cues, may progressively relegate control of movement to the intact motor areas, enabling PD subjects the acquisition of new skills and eventually facilitating structural and functional reorganization in the intact cortical areas. Canning (2005) affirms that since walking performance can be temporarily improved by manipulating attention, it may be that, with sufficient practice, improved walking performance could be learned in those with mild disease. Given that an experience-dependent plastic reorganisation depends on attention being paid by the recipient to the stimulation responsible for such changes (Racanzone et al 1993). Fisher et al (2004) demonstrated that MPTP (1 –methhyl- 4- phenyl-1,2,3,6-tetrahydropyridine) induced PD- like rats, treadmill walking for 30 days resulted in speed being recovered to the level of nonlesioned animals, along with increased synaptic occupancy of dopamine receptors in the brain. Therefore Mak and Hui (2008) suggest that if animal finding could be generalized to humans, training could have induced plastic changes in the human brain. The following discussion examines some of the possible strategies to overcome the four principal movement dysfunctions in PD subjects. The second part examines the possibility to integrate those movement strategies in performing three functional tasks (getting in and out of the bed, getting in and out of the chair and walking and turning within home).

VII1. Use of conscious and voluntary efforts to compensate the difficulty to use spontaneous and automatic movements;

PD subjects may learn to use voluntary movements and use attention function to compensate some of the difficulties linked to the generation of spontaneous activities during functional tasks. When basal ganglia are dysfunctional, as in PD, automaticity of movement is compromised and there is greater reliance on frontal-lobe attentional mechanism to control movements (Morris 2006). For example, during standing from sitting position PD subjects need to learn to draw their feet backwards, lean forward, using attentional system and voluntary muscle activity, before they stand up. Similarly walking trials could be performed with person using his or her internally generated instructions or mental images of long steps (Morris 1997). In able-bodied an internal focus of attention promotes conscious control of movements, thus interfering with automatic control processes which would normally control the movement. This is described by McNevin (2003), Totsika et al (2002) Wulf et al (2001) as a 'constrained action' hypothesis. In contrast, the finding on PD subjects by Canning (2005) has demonstrated an improved in walking performance by focusing attention on walking. This is because 'the reduced velocity and stride length in walking in PD are thought to reflect a loss of automaticity of well learned movements due to defective function of basal ganglia' (Morris 1994). Therefore it is not unexpected that instructions, which promote conscious control of the movement of walking, improve walking performances (Canning 2005). That is an external focus of attention is thought to allow the motor system to more naturally self organise, without interference from conscious control and so promote motor learning. However PD subjects with impaired attention may be unable to utilise attention system effectively to compensate an impaired automaticity. Given that 'the basal ganglia and limbic system particularly the afferent part of basal ganglia, which consists of caudate nucleus and putamen are probably involved in the selective component of attention' (Van Zomeren and Brouwer 1994). Furthermore despite intact attention function in some situation PD subjects may not be able to use attention function given 'the complexities of home and community environments and the multi-task nature of functional activities may interfere with one's ability to focus on attention and may limit the use of attentional strategies in certain situation' (Rochester et al 2005). They further suggest that attention strategies have a high cost in term of mental effort and fatigue as a result of using cognitive resources to generate the attentional cue. Therefore conscious voluntary movement, using attention function may help to compensate the absence of automatic involuntary movements; however in a complex environment other external cues like auditory or visual cues may be appropriate for facilitating functional tasks.

VII2. Strategies to overcome the difficulty to initiate and execute movements:

As mentioned earlier that the difficulty to initiate and execute movements result from a combination of dysfunctions; they include a breakdown of connection between BG to motor cortical areas; an impaired of neurotransmitter metabolism within basal ganglia neurons; and an attention dysfunction

The rhythmic auditory cues may help PD subject to minimise the difficulty to initiate and execute movements. Hömberg (1993) suggests that PD subjects are able to moderate their phasic alertness, that is, to reduce reaction time when they are forewarned by a stimulus preceding the "go" signal. The study on PD subjects by Rochester et al (2005) have demonstrated that use of auditory rhythmic cues in the context of the home environment and during functional activities leads to improvements in walking and mean step length. This study has provided information that not only PD subjects were able to integrate rhythmic auditory cues into a functional task immediately, but also they were able to improve usual functional activities within the home environment by using rhythmic auditory cues. Moreover auditory cues may be helpful to minimise gait freezing and help to improve walking in some individuals. Nieuwboer et al (1999) found that premature timing of tibialis anterior and gastrocnemius muscles occurs just before a gait freezing episode due to disturbance of central locomotor timing mechanisms and that the auditory cues provide one mechanism for overcoming this. Marchese et al (2000) also suggest that it is useful to incorporate external sensory stimuli in physical therapy protocols for moderately disabled patients with an aim of enabling them to learn new motor strategies. Fernandez del Olmo et al (2006) reported reduced movement variability in 9 people with PD after a 4 week program of daily gait training using auditory cues, and this finding correlated with changes in regional cerebral glucose utilisation as shown by positron emission tomography scans. Not only auditory stimulation but also visual stimulations help PD subjects to minimise their difficulty to initiate and execute movements. Sidaway et al (2006) found that 1month of gait training with visual cues establishes a lasting improvement in gait speed and step length while increasing the stability of the underlying motor control responsible for gait. Study carried out by Mak and Hui-Chan (2008) suggests that task-specific training strategy with audio-visual cues have produced more plastic changes in the brain than those of exercise training alone, leading to carry-over improvement to non-cued environment and to at least 2weeks after training ended.

Moreover Day et al (1984) suggest that although PD subjects are unable to make use of predictive action to reduce tracking error at the same extent as normal subjects, however they can reduce tracking error by using predictive strategy. This was demonstrated by Day et al (1984) that a reduction in the tracking lags to duration well below the reaction visual reaction time.

External cues may assist people with PD to move more easily because they utilise the intact premotor cortex of the brain rather than defective basal ganglia-supplementary motor area circuit to control movement (Goldberg 1985). However Morris (2000) suggests that the presence of external cue is not mandatory for activating neuronal networks in people with PD. PD subjects who are cognitively intact, simply focusing attention on crucial aspect of the movement that need to be controlled can be sufficient to activate movement with near normal speed and size (Morris et al 1996; Behrmanet et al 1998; Morris et al 1998). The distinction between attentional cueing strategies that must be generated internally through cognitive processes (such as thinking about the movement or size of a step) and external cues (auditory rhythmic tones) may therefore be important (Rochester et al 2005). The authors further suggest that a combination of cuing strategies may prove useful to address the wide variety of situations encountered and different level of ability. Therefore the external auditory and visual cue can minimise the difficulty to initiate an execute movements; however people with intact attention function may be able to minimise the inintialtion difficulties by focusing attention on the crucial aspect of the movement. Freezing episode where PD subject's feet remain attached to the floor is often results from initiation difficulty. This is mainly because of premature contraction of gastrocnemious producing planterflexion of the ankle instead of dorsiflexion. Some PD subjects can be able to minimise the episode of freezing by attending on dorsiflexion of the ankle during walking, or by practicing walking on the heel. Often during freezing PD subject use their voluntary effort to get rid of freezing, which reinforce freezing because the different muscle activities jump in to the higher frequency, including muscles of thigh and the trunk, whereas the initiation of walking by dorsiflexion of foot has not started. One strategy might be to stop walking and restart, either to start by lifting foot as if overcoming an obstacle, or to start by kicking with one foot.

Recently Mak and Hui-Chan (2008) investigated whether 4 weeks of audio-visual (AV) cued task-specific training could enhance sit-to-stand and whether the treatment effects could outlast the treatment period by two weeks. Fifty two subjects with PD completed the study. They were randomly allocated to receive 4 weeks of audio-visual cued task-specific training, conventional exercise, or no treatment (control).

- Audiovisual group were instructed to perform three tasks: sit-to-stand initiation, seat-off, and whole sit-to-stand. Visual cue was given on a computer screen with verbal command as auditory cue. Each task lasted two min, and was repeated once with 30-s rest in between. Training was given 20 min, 3 times a week for 4 weeks.
- The exercise group received conventional mobility and strengthening exercises for flexors and extensors of trunk, hip, knee and ankle followed by sot to stand practice. Training was 45 min, twice a week for 4 weeks. The same principal of progression was applied to both AV and exercise group, by increasing repetition number and reducing chair height for STS.
- The control group received no treatment.

Each subject was assessed before, at the end of 2 and 4 weeks of treatment, and 2 weeks after the treatment ended.

Result showed that the after of training, the audio-visual group significantly increase the peak horizontal velocity (13%, $P<0.01$) when compared with the exercise group. After 4 weeks of training, audio-visual group increased both peak horizontal and vertical velocities, respectably by 18% and 51%, and reduced the time to complete STS by 25%. These improvements were greater than those of the exercise group, who showed 8% and 20% increases respectably for peak horizontal and vertical velocities, and 10% decrease in movement time. Moreover the improvement of audio-visual cued group could be carried over to 2 weeks after treatment ended. The part-to-whole task specific training strategy with audio-visual cues have produced more plastic changes than exercise training alone, leading to carryover improvement to non-cued environment and to at least 2 weeks after training ended.

Therefore Mak and Hui-Chan (2008) have concluded from their study that both conventional exercise training and audio-visual cued task-specific training facilitated STS performances in PD subjects. However, cued task-specific training produced earlier and greater improvement than those with general exercise training. Moreover, AV cued task-specific training is recommended for patients with moderate severity of PD and without cognitive decline.

This randomised controlled trial provided concrete evidence for the use of audio-visual cued task-specific training can effectively overcome initiation difficulty while performing sit-to-stand in patients with PD.

It can be concluded that the difficulty to initiate and execute movement may be minimised by using different external cues, moreover PD subjects with intact cognitive function may minimise initiation and execution difficulty by focusing attention on the crucial aspect of the movement. Moreover the attention helps to produce internally generated movement, whereas different sensory cues dependent on external sensory stimulation. Therefore PD subjects may learn both the strategies to minimise the difficulty to initaiate movements.

VII3. Strategy to minimise the difficulty to perform large amplitude movements: Hömberg (1993) suggests that exercises involving large amplitude movements and truncal activities may facilitate rhythmic movement and therefore patient would be able to overcome miss-scaling of movements. Moreover, larger the amplitude of movement more it requires the number of interdependent and interrelated components of motor activities, increasing the difficulty to perform the entire frequency of movement. Often PD subjects use voluntary effort to overcome the difficulty. However instead of helping to perform large amplitude movement, the voluntary effort can provoke hastening. Therefore Hömberg (1993) suggests that optimal cueing frequencies must be found in individual patients in order to avoid 'hastening'. It is important that each PD subject has to identify optimal amplitude of movement during different physical activities. Moreover in case of 'hastening' resulting from large amplitude of movement, it is crucial to learn to stop and restart activity, instead of jumping into a higher frequency of movement. However Morris (1997) suggest that to overcome the difficulty to perform large amplitude movements walking trail can be performed while the physical therapist says 'long strides', 'think big' or 'step out' and other walking trials could be performed with the person using his or her own internally instruction or mental images of long steps. Moreover thinking of 'long stride' 'step out', and 'high steps' use attention function and facilitate internally generated movements, which can be effective to counteract the short steps and shuffling gaits. However given complicated environment condition and task demands many people may find it difficult use attentional strategies during walking. Therefore it is important that PD subjects learn to understand the optimal cuing frequency to avoid miscalling, at the same time practice large amplitude movement to ease the difficulty to perform large amplitude movements.

VII4.Strategies to overcome the difficulty to perform simultaneous and concurrent movements: Breakdown of simultaneous and concurrent movements during functional task into several simple acts may be an appropriate strategy. Strategies such as breaking down complex task into parts and focusing on unitask performance may need to be incorporated in the training program (Banks and Caird 1989), Formisano (1992). Hömberg (1993) also suggests that training of simple sequences during functional activities can improve motor control. For example to sit on a chair from walking may be disintegrated in to several simple acts, like reaching close to the chair, execute a 180° turn, and finally bend forward to sit down. Similarly to get out of the bed, subject turns on the side, swing the legs over the edge of the bed, push with the arms to sit on the edge of the bed. However according to Canning (2005) walking performance can be enhanced under duel task condition in people with moderate PD. Since walking performance under duel task condition is influenced by attention, specific instructions can be used in training to manipulate attention and enhance the performance of everyday duel-manual tasks in people with PD; for example, when walking is combined with an upper limb task, directing person's attention towards the task that is more critical for safety, i.e. the walking, may be the appropriate recommendation (Canning 2005). Therefore the tasks involved complicated concurrent movement may be simplified into several simple tasks to overcome difficulty to perform task; whereas duel tasks can be used as exercise to enhance walking performance.

Conclusion:

Four underlying movement dysfunctions are responsible for the difficulty to perform functional task in many PD subjects. These dysfunctions include absence of spontaneous movements, difficulty to initiate and execute movements, difficulty to perform large amplitude movements, and finally difficulty to perform complicated and concurrent movements. Integration of appropriate movement strategies during functional tasks can minimise these difficulties to a certain extent, in many PD subjects. These strategies include the use of conscious voluntary movements to counteract the absence of spontaneous movements; the use of external sensory cues as well as attention function to minimise the difficulty to initiate and execute movements. Moreover difficulty to perform large amplitude movement may be minimised by identifying an optimal length of movement. Complicated concurrent movements may be disintegrating in to several simple tasks. The duel tasks can be rehearsed, for the improvement of single task performance. The above movement dysfunction can have hindering effect to perform three functional tasks at home; - these tasks include, getting in and out of the bed, getting in and out of a chair, and walking and moving within their home. These task hindrances constitute the underlying factor for the progressive decline of autonomy and development of disability in many PD subjects. Therefore it can be assumed that the possibility to minimise the difficulties to perform these three tasks at home may uphold functional activity level and slow their disabling process. The next chapter examines some of the strategies to overcome the difficulty to perform the three functional asks.

Possible movement strategies to ease difficulty to perform the three functional tasks at home:

Introduction: Morris (2000) states that movement disorders are hallmark of PD and can severely compromise an individual's ability to perform well learned motor skills such as walking turning around, and transferring in and out of bed. Moreover Morris and Iansek (1997) affirm that although PD subjects can walk relatively quickly and easily in open spaces or very familiar environments, the slow stepped shuffling gait pattern that is so characteristic of the disease re-emerges in novel environments or congested spaces. Not only walking in congested space or within home environment constitute the part of movement difficulty in PD subjects but also other functional activities at home like getting in and out of the bed, getting in and out of a chair become progressively difficult. Each of these tasks has its specific organisational structure, which consists of a chain of interconnected and interdependent muscle activities. Moreover these organised activities are stored in the BG as programmed activities and the neural events within the BG enable these pre-programmed activities to be retrieved spontaneously. However despite the fact that these activities are retrieved spontaneously, a complex neural events take place to identify and prioritise a program among multiple programs, as well as to adapt and readapt movement strategy, that is suppresses one facilitates other in order to achieve the functional goal of the performer. Talland and Schwab (1964), Benecet al (1986), Benecke et al (1987) state that the defective basal ganglia compromise the person's ability to quickly shift from one mode of locomotion behaviour to another. The detrimental effect of these task difficulties is that they are responsible for the progressive loss of independence and development of disability in many PD subjects. Minimising of the task difficulties at home seems essential to uphold functional autonomy and to slow the development of disability. Therefore it is crucial to identify movement strategy to help PD subjects to minimise these task difficulties within their home environment. Ellis et al (2005) suggest that treatment administrated in the home environment may be necessary to allow direct instruction in the environment in which the behaviour change is desired. Nieuwboer et al (2001) found positive effects of a home PT (physiotherapy) for subjects with PD in the domains of gait, chair transfer, and bed mobility. Moreover functionally specific training is crucial for progressing functional status (Shumwau-Cook and Woollcott 1995). Furthermore task specific training seems particularly appropriate, given that movement disorders appear to be context dependent in PD subjects (Schultz et al 1995), and are most prominent for well-learned complex motor skills (Majsk et al 1998, Beneck et al 1987). However the evidence of the effects of training functional motor task comparing with the effect of training isolated movement is not available (Morris 2000). Given that PD symptoms results from a defective program controlled activities, it can therefore be assumed that the repeated practice of functional task at home may facilitate functional reorganisation in the intact neural circuits of the brain and progressively the program controlled activities might be relocated to the intact neural circuits of the brain. Jahanshahi et al (1995) state that externally cued movements are thought to bypass faulty basal ganglia-supplementary motor cortex pathways, and utilise cerebellar-premotor cortical pathways that may be intact in people with PD. In fact, motor learning is linked to cortical striatal plastic changes (Pisani et al 2005). The following discussion examines the possible strategies to PD subjects may learn to minimise difficulty to perform those tasks.

VIII 1.Getting out of the bed:

Getting in and out of bed requires one to perform several muscle actions in synchronised way, and for many PD subject it can become a very difficult and in extreme cases they require external help. One strategy can be to disintegrate these complicated muscle actions them into several simple actions. Moreover performing mental rehearsal of the sequences before starting can also alleviate the difficulty. Morris (2000) suggests the following strategy to get out of the bed:
- Shifting the pelvis toward the centre of the bed so that when turn is completed the body is not too close the edge.
- Turning the head
- Bringing the arms across the body in the direction of rolling
- Swinging the legs over the edge,
- pushing up, and
- Adjusting postural alignment to sit

VIII2. Getting out of a chair:

Standing from sitting (STS) moves body mass from a stable and supported sitting position to a relatively unstable and unsupported vertical position. The passage of flexed sitting position to extended standing position requires involvement of lower limb and trunk muscles. Moreover this passage from flexed sitting to extended standing position involves simultaneous and complex muscle activities work in a coordinated manner. Therefore it is clear that sit to stand requires strong lower limb and trunk muscles, relatively good balance function and most important is to be able to prioritise complex and simultaneous muscle activities in a synchronised manner. Difficulty to stand from sitting position for PD subjects is mainly due to difficulty to initiate movement and to perform complicated concurrent movements. In addition, along with difficulty to walk in a congested environment, difficulty to get in out of the bed, STS difficulty constitutes an important factor, which is responsible for the progressive loss of autonomy and development of disability in PD subjects. It is known that decrease in chair-raise time predicted future disability (Guralink et al 1995). In contrast improved STS performance could retard functional decline in peoples with PD (Mak and Hui-chan 2007). Before identifying an appropriate strategy of minimising sit to standing difficulty it is essential to examine the biomechanics of sit to stand.

VIII2a. Kinematic organisation of movement in sit to stand (STS):

STS requires translation of body mass in horizontal and vertical direction from a relatively stable sitting position with thighs and feet as base of support, to a period of relative instability when the thighs leave the seat and the feet become base of support (Carr and Shepherd 2004).

The transition of a secured standing from sitting requires strong and coordinated muscle work. Moving the body mass forward and upward is dependent on the strength and control of muscles of trunk as well as hip, knee, and ankle. Mak and Hui-Chan (2008) suggests that STS is a transitional task that involves propelling the body forward and upward from a wider (sitting) to narrower (stance) base. This passage from stable position to unstable position can augment risk of falls. Carr and Shepherd (2004) suggest that generating the angular and linear momentum to perform the horizontal vertical translatory moments of the body mass is potentially destabilising. According to Andriacchi et al (1980) and Berger et al (1988) standing up is one of the most mechanically demanding daily activities, requiring greater range of motion and higher moments of force at both hip and knee than gait and stair climbing. Moreover switching from one group of muscle action to another, as well as prioritising of one muscle action from among others involves selective attention. Selective attention reflects our capacity to select one stimulus source among others (Hochstenbach and Mulder 1999). It is clear then that sit to stand not only require strong muscle of lower limbs and trunk as well as good balance function but also cognitive function like selective attention plays crucial role in performing this task. In contrast the inability to stand up independently predisposes the individual to further decrease in muscle strength and physical fitness, and to adaptive soft tissue changes, particularly in soleus muscle, associated with disuse and physical inactivity. The difficulty link to stand from sitting position predisposes individual to minimise performing sit to stand and the fear of falling can have inhibiting effect on performing this task. Consequently many PD subjects tent to spend most of the day sitting. In addition The following discussion examines detailed movement analysis, which involves standing from sitting position.

Moreover the passage from wide base supported sitting to narrow based standing, which requires coordinated muscle action of both flexors and extensors of both lower limbs as well as the trunk. Therefore it is clear that STS involves synchronised actions of simultaneous muscle contractions.

For the ease of description, sit to stand can be divided into a first phase or pre-extension and a second phase or extension phase (Shepherd and Gentile 1994). In the first phase before initiation of standing from sitting position the feet are placed back and the subject leans forward. Feet placement is important in determining amount of extension force required by hip and knee to lift the body off from sitting position. Laboratory studies have shown that the further forward the feet, the greater the magnitude of hip flexion and the greater the velocity required to overcome the potential breaking force created by anterior foot position and move the body mass the additional distance forward(Vander Linden et al 1994). Vander Linden et al (1994), Shepherd and Koh (1996) suggest that anterior foot placement was shown to be associated with increase in peak hip moment of force and an increase in the duration of the extension phase, with muscle force therefore being sustained for a longer period then when the feet were back. This pre-extension phase is a spontaneous action generated by basal ganglia. Whereas in PD subject spontaneously placing feet back and brining trunk forward may be problematic mainly because of this placing of feet and bending of trunk forward. Instead feet remain forward compare to the vertical line that extends from the knee to the floor, and the subject fails to propel the body mass forward. It is clear then that the people with PD experience difficulty get out of a chair due to fact that their feet remain in front of the body, which requires greater hip moment of force as well as increase duration of extension phase. The organising difficulty in the first phrase can be responsible for the overall difficulty to get out of a chair.

The second phase is extension phase (Carr and Shepherd 2004), where vertical movement is brought about by extension at hips, knees, and ankle in a typical sequence of onsets, the knee starting to extend (at thigh-off) before the hip and ankle (Shepherd and Gentile 1994). In the extension phase the knee extension starts while the trunk is still flexing at the hip (Carr and Shepherd 2004). They affirm that this means that the body mass starts moving upward while it is still moving forward. This means while hip and trunk flexor are working to bring the trunk forward, the extension of the knees start to lift the thigh off the chair. It is evident from several studies that a timing relationship between the flexion of the trunk at the hip and onset of lower limb extension is a crucial feature in the movement organisation (Pai and Roger 1990, Schenkman et al 1990, Shepherd and Gentile 1994). Carr and Shepherd (2004) concluded from several studies that if patients do not rotate the upper segment through a range of 30 to 40°, at reasonable speed, and do not move body mass forward and upward without a pause between the two they will have to work harder to stand up. This movement organisation may be extremely difficult for PD subjects due to the difficulty to initiate movements, difficulty to switch one movement from one movement to another, and defective attention function.

VIII2b. Difficulty experience by PD subjects during STS:

Many PD subjects experience difficulty during spontaneous backward placing of feet and bringing body mass forward, while performing standing from sitting position. Whereas placing of feet backward and moving trunk forward before thigh-off are part of learned motor program, which are stored in the basal ganglia and can be retrieved spontaneously. The difficulty or unavailability of learned motor program PD subject will experience difficulty during first phase or pre-extension phase of STS. Moreover the first phase is the preparatory phase; this phase also acts as facilitator for the second phase. Therefore difficulty to perform the first phase of STS will add extra difficulty in performing second phase.

Moreover during extension phase several factors, which are linked to defective basal ganglia function, may be responsible for the difficulty to stand from sitting position. These factors include:
- difficulty to switch from one motor action to another,
- defective motor preparatory process,
- difficulty to initiate and execute movements,
- difficulty to perform simultaneous movements
- defective selective attention, and
- finally reduction in peak hip extension torque.

Switching from one group of muscle function to another can be extremely difficult for PD subjects. The body mass moves forward and then upward to stand from sitting which involve flexing of the trunk at the hip and then switching to extension of hips, knees and ankles. According to Mak and Hui-chan (2002) difficulty to initiate flexion of the trunk and then 'switch from flexion to extension is responsible the slowness of STS. Moreover markedly reduced peak hip extension torque (Mak and Hui-chan 2002) and a deficit in motor preparatory process could be causative factor (Rogers and Hui-chan 1988, Hui-Chan 1986).

During the second phase or the extension phase or the difficulty to initiate and execute movements, difficulty to perform simultaneous movements is responsible for the difficulty to stand from sitting.

Difficulty to initiate and execute movement may be responsible for the difficulty to initiate knee extension during thigh-off. Moreover once the thigh-off is achieved (as result of knee extension) initiation of hip extension starts in order to move the body upward. Therefore standing from sitting requires initiation and execution of several muscle groups. Evarts et al (1981) suggest that in PD time is prolonged both to initiate and to execute movements. A defect in motor preparatory process could be a causative factor for the slowness of STS (Chan 1986, Roger and Chan 1988). In addition one of the crucial moment of the second phase is that the knee extension starts (to lift off the thighs) while trunk is still moving forward. Once thigh-off the stool has attend to a certain extent, the moving forward of the trunk stops and extension at the level of hip and ankle, as well as static trunk extension starts. That is the hip extension starts while the knee is sill extending, and this simultaneous muscle function can be difficult if not impossible in some extreme cases for the PD subjects. Moreover performing simultaneous movements can be difficult due to defective selective attention function that results from defective basal ganglia function. Subjects with intact basal ganglia function able to prioritise concurrent movements and facilitate any one and suppress others using selective attention function and perform sit-to-stand without much difficulty. The PD subjects with degenerated BG and with impair selective attention function will perform STS slowly than people with intact selective attention function, and in extreme case they will need help get out of the chair.

Moreover muscle weakness that results from inactivity or reduced activity may compound to the overall difficulty to stand from sitting position. Mak and Hui-chan (2002), Mak et al (2003) suggest that the people with PD took longer time to complete STS then age matched controlled group, due to markedly reduced peak hip extension torque.

Given STS involves transferring body from relatively stable horizontal to vertical position, and this transferring of the body mass can be potentially destabilising. Therefore PD subjects with poor balance function will experience extra difficulty to perform STS.

It is clear then that several factors contribute to the difficulty during standing from sitting position in PD subjects. These factors include absence of spontaneous placing of feet backwards as well as bringing the trunk forward; difficult to initiate knee extension during thigh-off from the chair; difficulty to perform simultaneous knee extension and hip extension while moving the body upward. Overall difficulty of stranding from sitting position may compounded by poor balance function and weakness of lower limb muscles. It is therefore important to identify the strategy to overcome those difficulties.

VIII2c. Restore kinematic activity while standing from a sitting in PD subjects:

People with PD can learn to use conscious voluntary movement in the absence of spontaneous pulling of feet backward and leaning forward of the trunk. Simultaneous complicated movements like leaning forward and extension of knee can be disintegrated in several simple acts. Moreover delay in initiation of movement may be minimised by using external sensory cues. Audio-visual cues which give 'preparatory' single before PD subjects initiate sit-to-stand, may improve their performance compare to no-cued situation. AV cues given as advance information could have heightened patients' attention to facilitate movement execution. External cued movements are thought to bypass faulty basal ganglia-supplementary motor cortex pathways, and to utilise cerebellar-premotor cortical pathways that might be intact in PD (Jahashahi et al 1995).

In addition during sit-to-stand using audiovisual cues, the selective attention to audiovisual cues may enhance explicit learning leading to declarative memory of the movement sequence (Kelly et al 2004). With repetitive sit-to-stand practice, this declarative knowledge could have translated into procedural knowledge (Pasual-Leon et al 1993). Declarative or explicit memory involves with factual knowledge, and procedural or implicit memory deals with knowledge on how to perform activities (Squire et al 1993). So, the selection of the most adequate motor action involves the explicit memory system, whereas the performance of the action involves implicit memory system (Hochstenbach and Mulder 1999). Mak and Hui-Chan (2008) found that after 2 weeks of AV cued-training subjects with PD were able to produce better STS initiation and execution even in the absence of AV cues. Therefore it is clear that task-specific AV-cued training enhances the transformation of explicit knowledge into implicit knowledge leading to long-term improvement of function.

The complicated muscle action of sit to stand can be broken down in to several sequences, which is proposed by (Morris 2000):

- Shifting body forward so that the buttocks are close to the edge of the chair,
- Placing the feet on the floor so that heels are well back
- Leaning the trunk forward, and
- Standing up quickly while thinking of leaning "forward and up" in and arc of movement.

VIII2d Sitting on a chair from walking:

When approaching a chair with the intention of turning around to sit down, the person's foot steps are dramatically reduced in size and speed, and freezing occurs prior to and during the turning maneuver. Morris (2000) proposes to break prehension movements down in to separate parts like terminating the straight-line walking sequence and performing the turning and sitting down components separately and concentrate on performing each component separately. Moreover during walking and sit on a chair, PD subject might benefit by planning and mentally rehearsing the procedure (Morris 2000). For example walk to sit on a chair can break down into sequences of 3 actions

- First of all the subject walks as close as possible to the chair,
- Then turn round so that the chair is behind the subject, and
- Finally bent forward (flexion of hips, knees, and trunk) to sit down.

Conclusion:

STS is an important function task of daily living and many PD subjects may find it extremely difficult to perform this task. It involves transfer of the body mass from a relative stable horizontal position to an unstable vertical position. This transformation of body mass involves leaning forward of the trunk, extension of the knee, and hips. Therefore it is clear that one needs strong muscle force of lower limb muscles, and good balance function to perform effectively STS function. STS can be divided into two distinct phases, pre-extension phase, and extension phase. Pre-extension phase consists of pulling feet backward and bringing the trunk forward; whereas extension phase consists of moving the body forward and upward. Pre-extension phase involves initiation and execution of movements as well as automatic background movements, whereas extension phase consists of simultaneous flexion of trunk and extension of the knees; as well as simultaneous extension of both knees, both hips and the trunk. Difficulty to initiate and execute movements, absence of automatic background movements, and difficulty to perform simultaneous movements, which may be underlying factors for standing difficulty from sitting position in PD subjects. Freezing and festinaion can occur while sitting on a chair from walking. Therefore this complex movement can be divided in to several simple acts.

VIII3. Walking and turning difficulty in PD:

Walking difficulty is an early sign in PD. As the disease progresses there may be progressive deterioration of walking capacity with loss of autonomy, and eventual development of disability in PD subjects. Walking is a complex whole-body action that requires the cooperation of the both legs and coordination of a large number of muscles and joints to function together (Carr and Shepherd 2004).

Parkinson gait is characterised by short-stepped, shuffling gait, with episodes of festination and freezing. Moreover these gait characteristics are more prominent in a congested environment for example within home. Because walking within home consists of walking and turning, which needs frequent adaptations and adjustments. Moreover this difficulty of moving within home contribute to the progressive decline of activity level and development of disability in many PD subjects; it therefore important that PD subjects learnt to overcome walking and turning difficulty within home. The following discussion analyse the biomechanical aspects of human walking, walking and turning difficulty in PD subjects.

VIII3 a. Kinematic motor organisation in walking:

Smooth walking is assured by combination of muscle activities, intact sensory function, as well as ability to balance in standing position. Moreover cognitive function like attention plays important role during walking. Muscle activities consist of static muscle work as well as dynamic muscle work. While one group of muscle works statically to assure stability of joint, the others work dynamically to provide propulsion of the limb to move the body forward. In fact static and dynamic muscle function along with different sensory functions enables one to maintain upright position and enable one to adapt and adjust in constant changing position of body as well as constant change of environment. According to Carr and Shepherd (2004) many structural and physiological elements or components cooperate to produce coordinated walking in a changing environment. In addition coordinated walking is obtained 'by linking muscles and joints so that they act together as a single unite or synergy, thus simplifying the coordination of movement' (Bernstein 1967). Different sensory systems also function to facilitate smooth walking. Sensory system includes proprioception and exterioception, where proprioception is superficial sensation and deep sensation from different joints of lower limb. Exterioception includes visual, auditory, and vestibular sensation. Carr and Shepherd (2004) suggest that sensory input in general and visual input in particular provide information that makes it possible for us to walk in varied, cluttered environment and uneven terrains. However as sensory function has its diverse aspects (e.g. superficial and deep sensation, visual and proprioception) in case of impairment of one aspect of sensory function, the other sensory function compensate that loss, that enable one to walk despite loss of one of the sensory function. For example impaired visual sensation in case of blindness one can continue to walk, in which case the acuity other sensory functions increase in order to compensate loss of visual sensation. Similarly loss of propioception can be compensated by visual sensation. Therefore it is clear that walking performance requires adequate muscle force, intact sensory, cognitive as well as intact balance function, and impairment of any of these functions may severely jeopardy individual's ability to walk.

Using voluntary and involuntary muscle function, sensory function, intact balance function, bilateral alternative movements of both lower limbs enable human to walk. Moreover bilateral alternative movements of lower limbs produce a stance phase and a swing phase; in stance phase the body is supported by one leg, while the other leg swings to move the body forward. According Carr and Shefherd (2004) the gait cycle includes a stance phase (approximately 60%) and a swing phase (approximately 40%). The stance phase can be further subdivided into weight acceptance, mid-stance and push-off, while swing is divided into lift-off (early swing) and reach (late swing) (Winter 1987). In-between stance and swing phase, there are two brief period of double support phases. The duration of double support time may increase with aging; that is as the time spent in double support increases people walk slower, and with increase of velocity of walking time spent in double support reduces. Therefore it is clear that good muscle and sensory functions are essential for smooth walking performance. Moreover balance reaction is also an important factor for facilitate smooth performance of gait cycle. It is the ability to balance the body mass relative to the base of support that enables us to perform everyday actions, (including walking) effectively and efficiently (Carr and Shepherd 2004). They further state that apart from double support period, the body is in a potentially unstable state. Safe foot clearance and foot contacts are, therefore essential to rebalancing the body mass during double support (Winter et al 1987). With aging process as balance skill impairs, many elderly people compensate by increasing double support phase, as well as widening the base of support or the distance between two feet.

VIII3b. Analysis of Kinematic organisation in walking:

Kinematic variables provide information about angular displacements, paths of the body parts and the centre of body mass (CBM), with angular and linier velocities and accelerations (Carr and Shepherd 2006). Normally individual variations in the magnitude of angular displacement are relatively small, with the greatest variances occurring in the less obvious movements of ankle and foot (Sutherland et al 1994). Carr and Shepherd (2006) describe that the mass of the upper body, including pelvis and trunk, responds to the needs of the individual to advance the lower limb and to transfer body weight from one supporting limb to other. For example, the pelvis (moving at the hip joints and joints of the lumbar spine) rotates, tilts, and shifts laterally, governed by such factors as muscle length and length of stride. Shoulders rotate and arm swing out of phase with displacement of pelvis and leg. Moreover while one group of muscles work dynamically the other work statically to assure smooth walking. During stance phase the body weight is supported by one leg and this supporting is maintained by static work of muscles of trunk, pelvis and lower limb, at the same time muscles of the other side of the body work dynamically to propel the limb forward. The movements of the trunk, pelvis as well as both lower limbs and upper limbs are automatic and require very little voluntary effort. In fact walking skill is acquired in early stage of life using conscious and voluntary activities, in this acquisition process attention function plays important role. Progressively walking skills are relegated to basal ganglia. The walking skills are then stored as memory in the basal ganglia, which can be retrieved when needed. The possibility of store and retrieve walking skills in basal ganglia enables one to walk automatically without using conscious and voluntary effort. Not only walking skills but other motor skills also undergo this storing and retrieving process, and this process constitute the underlying factor for the skill acquisition. With degeneration of basal ganglia this storing and retrieving process of motor skills are impaired, resulting in walking difficulty.

The loss of dopamine-producing cells in the substantia nigra progresses over time, gait disorders become more severe and variable in their presentation in the advance stage of the disease (Morris et al 1994). As a result of basal ganglia dysfunction people with Parkinson's disease experience difficulty to initiate and execute movement, difficulty to perform large amplitude movement, difficulty to perform simultaneous movements and absence of automatic background movements. These movement dysfunctions are mainly responsible for the waking difficulty in PD subjects. According to Forssberg (1992) the major requirements for successful walking are:

- (1) Support body mass by lower limbs
- (2) Propulsion of body in intended direction
- (3) the production of a basic locomotion rhythm
- (4) the balance control of the moving body
- (5) Flexibility, i.e. the ability to adapt the movement to changing environmental demands and goal.

When the above sequences are analysed in PD subjects it is observed that:

- (1) <u>Support of body mass by lower limbs</u> remains intact in PD subjects, unless in advance stage of the disease when due to inactivity there is structural and functional change of soft tissues and joints of lower limb.
- (2) <u>Propulsion of body in intended direction:</u> PD subjects often experience difficulty to propel body in the intended direction, mainly due to difficulty to initiate and execute movements. Moreover frizzing episodes will make it extra difficult for the propultion of the body in intended direction.
- (3) <u>The production of basic locomotion rhythm</u> is impaired mainly due to rigidity of muscles. Moreover due to absence of automatic background movement PD subject will unable to produce basic locomotion rhythm. Instead PD subjects walk like a rigid block, with diminution or absence of dissociation between pelvic and pectoral girdles, as well as diminution or absence of arm swing and dorsiflexion of feet.
- (4) <u>Balance control of the moving body:</u> Balance reaction remains intact in PD; however falls and balance disturbance is common in PD. A neurotransmitter disturbance associated with basal ganglia degeneration may contribute to balance impairment, moreover muscle rigidity and later in the disease process muscle weakness may perturb balance function.
- (5) <u>Flexibility, i.e. the ability to adapt the movement to changing environmental demands and goal:</u> The ability to adapt and adjust with home or in a congested environment remains most difficult part of walking for the PD subjects. Often PD subjects can walk perfectly in an open space, the PD symptoms like reduced speed and step amplitude, increased

stepping frequency and, in some cases festination and freezing appear with in home environment. This may be due to difficulty to switch from one movement to another and due to difficulty to perform simultaneous movements.

VIII3c Walking difficulty in PD:

Morris et al (1994) states that gait disturbance in PD is characterised reduced speed and step amplitude, increased stepping frequency and, in some cases festination and freezing. According to Murray et al (1997) walking in PD is characteristically slow, short stepped, and shuffling, with reduced arm swing and often stooped posture. Canning et al (2006) suggest that four motor impairments likely to contribute to walking capacity, which are hypokinesia during walking (that is reduced speed and amplitude of movement), hypokinesia during turning, automaticity, and muscle strength.

The clinical observation reveals that difficulty of walking includes initiation and termination difficulty, along with shortened footsteps and ground clearance difficulty. Difficulty to initiate and execute movement, absence of automatic and background movements, difficulty to perform large amplitude movements are added to the gait difficulty in PD subjects.

However Morris et al (1994) suggest that the primary gait deficit in PD is mainly inability to generate sufficient amplitude of movement. According to Huxham et al (2008) the motor command governing walking may be normal, but the dysfunctional basal ganglia are unable to maintain or match the required amplitude of movement. Therefore Morris et al (1994) advocate that increasing step amplitude should be the primary goal of therapy intended to normalize gait.

Gait difficulty leading to inactivity may result in musculoskeletal impairments such as weakness, reduces flexibility of joints and their eventual deformity. Inactivity may also be responsible for the cardiopulmonary impairment such as reduced aerobic capacity. Walking dysfunction is common in neurologically impaired individuals arising not only from the impairment associated with the lesion but also from secondary cardiovascular and musculoskeletal consequence of disuses and physical inactivity. These secondary impairments may further deteriorate the gait performance in PD subjects. In addition typical characteristic of Parkinsonian walking is more prominent in a congested environment for example inside home, and it seems walking difficulty within home environment contribute to progressive deterioration of walking capacity. The underlying reason may be that walking in a congested environment consists of walking and turning, which require frequent adapting and adjusting of step amplitude.

Turning difficulty in PD: Stack et al (2006), Morris and Iansek (1997) affirm that turning during locomotion is typically problematic in the early and middle stage of the disease progression and can be associated with trips and falls, and freezing episodes. The efficiency and safety of turning of normal turning are often lost in people with PD (Huxam et al 2008). They further suggest that differences in adjustment of step time to turn may reflect impaired locomotor turning control in subjects with PD during challenging gait tasks; for example walking in a congested environment. Moreover turning difficulty is a frequent component of gait disturbance and functional disability in people with PD (Nieuwboer et al 1998). Turning occurs frequently in all daily actions performed while walking (Huxam et al 2008). As many as five turns are needed in every 10m within the home (Sedgman et al 2004). Often many PD subjects can walk easily without much difficulty in a straight line, and the difficulty often arises during turning. Therefore it is important that PD subject learn to walk as well as to turn.

Huxam et al (2008) conducted a randomised controlled trial in 10 people with PD and 10 age, gender – and height matched control subjects. In the study they examined the spatiotemporal characteristic footstep adjustment used to turn 60 and 120 degrees were examined in using three-dimensional motion analysis. Control subjects used a recognizable pattern of spatial and temporal footstep modulations to turn. Participants with PD demonstrated significant differences in almost all variables. They (1) failed to turn as far as their peers; (2) showed a similar but scaled-down pattern of spatial adjustment to turn; (3) used sorter strides when walking, with exaggerated reduction when turning; (4) demonstrated small significant temporal differences in step time adjustments. Therefore the study concluded that people with PD were unable to turn as effectively as controls despite normal patterning of foot step adjustments. Strong spatial differences as baseline become more marked when turning, especially in the large turn. Excessive stride length reduction in large turns by subjects with PD may contribute to turning difficulty in susceptible individuals. Altered step time adjustments in larger turn may suggest the timing control of gait in PD is impaired under challenging condition.

Another study by Huxham (2006) using 3-dimensional motion analysis, measured self-paced 60° turns during walking in people with PD compared with young and older adults without impairments. Those with PD showed shorter step length and reduced axial rotation at the pelvis as well as diminished counter-balancing activity at the thorax, even for this relatively small turning angle. It is clear than that walking difficulties along with turning difficulty exaggerate difficulty to move within the home environment. Therefore it is important for PD subjects to learn strategies to overcome difficulty to walk and turn within home environment.

Role of attention in walking:

Attention forms an important part of the cognitive system. Zomeren and Brower (1994) define attention as a cognitive state characterised by a selective bias for processing certain internal and external stimuli. They further suggest that the important aspects of attention in this respect are selectivity, intensity, and its dynamic character. According to Theeuwis (1992) attention is essential to the correct perception of conjunctions, though unattended features are often conjoined prior to their conscious perception. This top down feature is capable of utilizing past experience and contextual information. The attention system has an important role to perform in registering and processing all information received. An impaired capacity of attention can have serious consequences on neural recovery and attaining functional autonomy. Moreover although different functional tasks are the result of spontaneous retrieving of learned movement, nevertheless selective attention plays an important role in organising and prioritising the complex concurrent movements of a given task into synchronised manner. The following discussion examines briefly the different aspects of attention, looking at the part of the brain responsible for the attention function, as well as its importance for neural recovery and reacquisition of functional activity.

Van Zomeren and Brouwer (1994) describe the attention system as having four distinct parts, comprising selective, focused, divided and sustained attention. These distinctive features of the system of attention are explained as follows:

3. Selective attention reflects our capacity to distinguish one source of stimulus from another.
4. Focused attention enables us to direct the attention to the main aspect of a task without being distracted by irrelevant stimuli.
5. Divided attention reflects our capacity to shift between several input sources or tasks and to do two or more things simultaneously.

Sustained attention reflects the ability to concentrate on a given task over long and generally unbroken periods of time without a substantial decline or large fluctuation in the performance.

Selective attention plays important role in prioritising one group of muscle activity, while inhibiting other during walking and turning or walking in changing environment.

VIII

Strategies to Minimise Walking and Turning Difficulties in PD Subject

VIII 3d 1Use attention strategy:

PD subjects with gait hypokinesia (slowness of walking) divert their attention from their footsteps to a second task such as carrying a tray with drinks or talking the stride length and gait speed immediately show marked reductions (Morris et al 1996; Bond et al 2000; and Morris et al 2000). Therefore Morris et al (1996) and Bond et al (2000) propose that avoiding duel task performance during gait helps people to maintain long strides during walking. Attentional strategies such as focusing attention on the key aspects of the gait pattern requiring improvement, avoiding the performance of a secondary motor or cognitive task that may compromise safety during gait, and breaking down long or complex locomotor sequences into component parts and concentrating on the performance of each part can enable people to walk more easily (Morris 2000; Rochester et al 2004). However Cunning (2005) suggests that avoid performing duel task is impractical in many circumstances and would limit physical activity in those with mild to moderate disease. The study by Canning (2005) has demonstrated that walking performance was temporarily improved in dual task condition. The author suggests that since walking performance under duel-tasks conditions is influenced by attention, specific instructions can be used in training to manipulate attention walking performance; for example, when walking is combined with a upper limb task directing the person's attention towards that is more critical for safety, i.e. the walking, may be the appropriate recommendation. Therefore it is important to disintegrate complicated concurrent tasks into several simple tasks, for example walking and turning may be separated into walking in straight line, and then turning; whereas duel-task during walking may be used as therapy to enhance walking; for example, carrying a tray and walking.

VIII 3d 2 Creating a mental maps to improve gait performance:

It may be useful for the Parkinson subjects to learn to create a mental representation of the trajectory to be covered each time each time prior to start walking. Morris et al (1997) suggest that preparing in advance for forthcoming by using mental rehearsal and visualization might also be benefit. One explanation might be that the subjects with Parkinson's disease are able to construct internal model of the task, they appear to have difficulty in forming a dynamic internal model of their own movements. As a result, they may not be able to make use of predictive action to reduce tracking error substantially to the same extent as is evident in the normal subjects (Day et al 1984). Therefore during walking, when a sudden change in the direction is needed for example avoiding furniture or to turn on the corridor, Parkinson subjects find it difficult to change the direction spontaneously, they either change direction brusquely, or often get stuck in a place. Creating a mental map regarding the distance and the turning that have to be covered during each functional activity may help to reduce tracking error. Moreover strategy to use mental map facilitate internally generated response, which 'uses an attentional strategy and requires planning and feed forward motor control' (Gueye et al 1998). However this approach of creating mental map to overcome tracking error may be useful only in a familiar environment and people with cognitive impairment especially impaired executive function will face extra difficulty to create a mental map.

Therefore crating a mental map (cognitive map) of the entire trajectory before starting any functional activity, like getting out of the bed to go the toilet, getting out of a chair and go to the other room or the kitchen and eventually sit on a chair may help PD subject to minimise tracking error and reduce festinating and freezing episodes.

VIII 3d 3Attention strategy:

Attentional strategy such as focusing attention on the key aspect of the gait pattern requiring improvement, avoiding the performance of a secondary motor or cognitive task that may compromise safety during gait (Morris 2006).
- Breaking down long complex locomotor sequences into component parts and concentrating on the performance of each part can enable people to walk more easily (Morris 2000; Rochester 2004).

VIII 3d 4.Strategy to integrate auditory cues:

Auditory cues that aim to normalise locomotor timing such as provided by a musical beat or rhythmical chanting can help some people move more easily (McIntosh et al 1997; Thaut et al 1996; Nieuwboer et al 1999, Rochester et al 2005; Burleigh et al 1997). Nieuwboer et al (1999) found that premature timing of the tibialis anterior and gastrocnemius muscles occurs just before a gait freezing episode due to a disturbance of central locomotor timing mechanisms and auditory cues provide one mechanism for overcoming this. Moreover difficulty to initiate movement during walking can be minimized or motor readiness can be improved if PD subjects are forewarned with an auditory stimulation. According to Hömberg (1993) PD subjects are able to moderate their phasic alertness, that is, to reduce reaction times when they are forewarned by a stimulus preceding the 'go' signal.

Rochester et al (2005) investigated the effect of external rhythmic cues (auditory and visual) on walking during functional task in homes of people with PD. They hypothesized that the use of an external (rhythmic) cue during the functional task would reduce gait interference because it demanded less attention than when performing task with no cue, which requires someone to use cognitive processes to divide attention between tasks. In this research the change in walking speed was achieved by an increase in step length, because there were no changes in step frequencies.

Fernandez del Olmo et al (2006) reported that reduced movement variability in 9 people with PD after 4 weeks program of daily gait training using auditory cues, and this finding correlated with regional cerebral glucose utilization as shown by position emission tomography scans. However it is important that PD subjects are able to integrate the auditory stimulation strategy with in the home environment, because there is no evidence that improved performances at the therapy department can be generalized in a more complicated home environment. Rochester et al (2005) calculated walking speed, step frequency, and step amplitude in PD subjects, the participants used auditory cues within home environment; however the value obtained were generally lower than other results in laboratory situation. Therefore they suggest that the results in home environment may represent the added influence of complex home environment.

Summary of the strategies to minimise walking difficulties:

- use visual and verbal cues during walking (counting, look at an object above the eye level, a wall clock for example).
- Use of internally generated instructions or mental image of long steps during walking (Morris and Iansek 1997).
- Walking on the heel to avoid episode of freezing.
- To overcome episode of freezing during turns, people with PD can be trained to concentrate on turning in a large arc of movement, using full body movements, rather than focusing on rapid switching directions (Yekutiel et al 1991)
- use 'clock turn' strategy for turning while on a small space, which consists of person stands on the spot and then consciously thinks of stepping with the right foot then the left to the relevant position for the task (eg, to make a 180° turn, step to 12 o'clock, 3 o'clock, and 6 o'clock). Attention is directed to lifting the feet clear in a deliberate stepping action, rather than shuffling and swiveling around (Kirkwood et al 1997).

- Use conscious, voluntary movement to compensate the absence of background involuntary movements.
- Use visual and verbal cues to bypass involvement of basal ganglia in order to overcome difficulty to initiate and execute movement.
- Optimal length of movement has to be identified in order to avoid difficulty to perform large amplitude movements.
- Learn to disintegrate simultaneous tasks into several simple tasks during functional activities

Learn to use to create mental map before each functional activity.

Some of the strategies to minimise the difficulty to perform three functional tasks at home:

1. Getting in and out of the bed:

<u>To get out of the bed PD subjects practice the following sequences:</u>
- Shift the pelvis toward the centre of the bed so that when turn is completed the body is not too close the edge.
- Bend the knees
- Turn the head
- Bring the arms across the body in the direction of rolling
- Swing the legs over the edge,
- Push up, and
- Adjusting postural alignment to sit (Morris 2000)

Plan and mentally rehearse the sequences each time before starting.

<u>Getting in to the bed:</u>
- Reach close to the bed
- Turn round to sit on the bed
- Move the buttocks towards the middle of the bed so that the back of the knees touch the edge of the bed.
- Finally lie on the side and pull the feet on the bed

Plan and mentally rehearse the sequences each time before starting.

2. Get in and out of a chair:

<u>Getting in to a chair:</u>

During walking and sit on a chair, PD subject might benefit by planning and mentally rehearsing the procedure for terminating the straight-line walking sequence and performing the turning and sitting down components separately (Morris 2000).

- First of all the subject reaches as close as possible to the chair,
- Then turn round so that the chair is behind the subject, and
- Finally bent forward to sit down.

Getting out of chair:

It is necessary to sequence 4 actions:

- Shift body forward so that the buttocks are close to the edge of the chair,
- Place the feet on the floor so that heels are well back
- Lean forward, and
- Stand up quickly while thinking of leaning "forward and up" in and arc of movement (Morris 2000).

3. Walking and turning:

<u>Walking:</u>

- Create a mental map (cognitive map) of the entire trajectory before start walking like go to the other room or the kitchen.
- Attentional strategy such as focusing attention on the key aspect of the gait pattern requiring improvement, avoiding the performance of a secondary motor or cognitive task that may compromise safety during gait (Morris 2006).
- Breaking down long complex locomotor sequences into component parts and concentrating on the performance of each part can enable people to walk more easily (Morris 2000; Rochester 2004), for example turning and walking are done separately, or sitting and walking are done separately.
- Use visual and verbal cues during walking (counting, look at an object above the eye level, a wall clock for example).
- Use of internally generated instructions or mental image of long steps during walking (Morris and Iansek 1997).

- Incase of freezing, learn to stop, lean back ward, and restart walking, instead of forcing to try to move forward (often PD subjects find it convenient to restart by giving a kick, others restart by lifting one foot as if overcoming little obasacle)

<u>Turning:</u>
- Concentrate on turning in a large arc of movement, using full body movements, rather than focusing on rapid switching directions (Yekutiel et al 1991)
- Use 'clock turn' strategy for turning while on a small space, which consists of person stands on the spot and then consciously thinks of stepping with the right foot then the left to the relevant position for the task (e.g., to make a 180° turn, step to 12 o'clock, 3 o'clock, and 6 o'clock). Attention is directed to lifting the feet clear in a deliberate stepping action, rather than shuffling and swiveling around (Kirkwood et al 1997).

IX Secondary factors, which contribute to the reduced activity level in PD subjects:

The previous discussion has concentrated mainly on different movement dysfunctions and the possible strategies to overcome those movement dysfunctions. However BG degeneration may be responsible for a wide spread cognitive and behavioural dysfunctions. Sensory, emotional and perceptual signs are also observed in some individuals (Bhatia and Marsden 1994). Resting tremor, rigidity, and later in the disease process, postural instability falls are associated characteristic of PD (Jankovic and Tolsa1988, Jankovic et al 2001). Moreover these associated dysfunctions may have profound repercussion on functional activity level; and therefore, a physical intervention strategy to overcome movement dysfunction may have very limited impact on the activity level in PD subjects with severe cognitive, behaviour dysfunction and other associated dysfunctions.

IX 1. Structural and functional changes of different tissues contributing to further reduction of the activity level:

The reduced activity level in PD subjects may have a negative repercussion of the structure and function of different tissues around the joint. Impairments of body structure and body function are associated with limitation in activities such as walking in the home and community, moving from a lying to sitting to standing position, and turning (Stack et al 2006). These impairments of structure and function of different tissues may further aggravate difficulty to perform different functional tasks. Moreover changes of structures and function of different tissues may eventually alter postural and balance reaction in PD subject minimising further their activity level. The following discussion will examine repercussions of reduced activity level on structures and functions of muscles, bone, ligament, and cartilage. Different aerobic activities strengthening exercise may help to uphold the structure and functional properties of different tissues. The following discussion examines the structures and functions of muscles and other non-contractile and bone and the consequences of inactivity.

IX 2 Change in muscle:

<u>The effects of inactivity on muscles:</u> Inactivity and suboptimal activity may be responsible for muscle atrophy and muscle weakness. The people with PD have more rapid drop in physical activity levels than age matched controlled subjects (Fertle et al 1993). The reduced activity level leading to stress deprivation of muscles may be responsible for the production of weakness of different muscles of the lower limb. According to Laumonnier and Belton (2000) the diminution of muscle force in PD is not directly linked to the disease process but due to under use of different muscles. They further suggest that although dynamic (isotonic) muscle force is often impaired, but static (isometric) muscle force is conserved for long time in PD. It is clear then that muscle weakness added to the other movement dysfunctions caused by BG degeneration may contribute to further reduction in activity level in PD. The following discussion reviews the underlying factors responsible for muscle weakness.

According to Carr and Shepherd (2004) weakness and fatigability of muscles can arise secondary from disuse, especially if person spends much of the day sitting down. In a sedentary situation the secondary changes are particularly evident in antigravity postural muscles since their previous roles are no longer practised in this situation. The quadriceps atrophy occurs as early as 3 days after immobilisation in normal individuals (Lindboe and Platou 1984). Halkjae-Kristensen and Ingeman-Hansen (1985) affirm that 30% reduction the cross-section area of quadriceps muscle fibres occurs within one month of immobilisation. Disuse atrophy of muscles may accompany their adaptive shortening. In contrast physical training has been found to increase the cross-section area of the muscle fibres accounting for the increase in muscle bulk and strength (Arvidson et al 1984; Eriksson and Häggmark 1979; Häggmark et al 1981; Thorstensson et al 1977). The potential of adult skeletal muscle fibres to change their biomechanical properties in response to functional demands is remarkable (Diez et al 1986).

Impaired motor drive can be a result of the lesion and disuse (McComas 1994); and an impaired motor drive may be responsible for the minimising muscle use. Moreover McComas et al (1995) suggest that disuse accentuates muscle fatigue by reducing the ability of motor centres to recruit motor neurons maximally. Furthermore lack of muscle activity and of joint movement results in adaptive anatomical, mechanical, and functional changes to the neural and muscular system, which include loss of functional motor units (McComas 1994).

According to Carr and Shepherd (2002) these changes include change of muscle fibre type, physiological change in muscle fibres and change in muscle metabolism, and increased muscle stiffness. Muscles subjected to prolonged positioning at a short length, and which are rarely exposed to active and passive stretch, undergo change in cross-bridge connection and become shorter (develop contractures) and stiffer (Carr and Shepherd 2002). Changes in connective tissue contribute both to stiffness and contracture (William et al 1988), since water loss and collagen deposition also occur in response to disuse (Carey and Burghardt 1993). Increase stiffness is also found in the absence of contracture (Malouin et al 1997). Clinical and laboratory tests have demonstrated the functional interference by increased stiffness (Sinkjaer and Magnussen1994). Reduced activity level in PD subject may be responsible for the stress deprivation of muscles, which in turn facilitates the development of muscle stiffness and muscle contracture, compounding the task difficulties. Postural muscles with a large proportion of slow twitch fibres (e.g. soleus) may develop stiffness due to lack of activity, and stiffness and contracture of soleus can have significant functional effects, interfering with walking, standing up and balancing in standing Carr and Sheferd (2004)

IX 3 Prevention of muscle weakness in PD:

Carr and Shepherd (2000) suggest that skilled motor performance requires:

V. Each muscle involve in the generation of peak force at the length appropriate to the action,
VI. This force has to be graded and timed so synergic muscle activity is controlled for task and context,
VII. The force has to be sustained over sufficient period of time.
VIII. The peak forces must be generated fast enough to meet environmental task demands such as increasing walking speed.

Although muscle weakness contributes to the deterioration of activity level, however muscle strengthening itself is not sufficient for improving functional activity level in Parkinson subjects, since movement dysfunctions that result from basal ganglia degeneration are the principal attribute to reduce activity level in PD.

IX 3a Task specific training to prevent deterioration of muscle function:

Individual muscle strengthening and aerobic exercise are often used as therapeutic approach to thwart movement difficulty in PD subjects. However despite training for strengthen individual muscle strength, PD subjects continue to experience movement difficulties, this is mainly because strengthening muscle may not able to minimize movement difficulties. In contrast task specific activities seem to be more effective, because in one hand they directly address the functional difficulties of PD on the other hand repetitive use those tasks during daily activities may slow decline of functional status. The following discussion the effect of exercise on muscles, appropriateness of task specific training, and finally the importance of repetition of tasks on long-term improvement of function is also discussed.

The neuromuscular adaptation associated with muscle strengthening in the able-bodied is due to neural adaptations to neural drive, which are both quantitative (increase neural drive to the target muscles) and qualitative (reduced co-contraction and improve coordination among synergists) (Hakkinen and Komi 1983; Rutherford and Jones 1986; carolan Caarelli 1992; Yue and Cole 1992). Moreover different exercises to improve muscle force will enhance muscle excitation capacity, improve rate of recruitment of motor neuron pool, capacity to inhabit agonist muscles, motor unit activation and synchronization and motor firing pattern will also be ameliorated (Hakkinen and Komi 1983, Sale 1987). Furthermore different strengthening training enhance stimulation of metabolic, mechanical and structural muscle fiber changes that result in larger and stronger muscles due to an increase in actin and myocin protein filaments (Sale 1987; Thepaut-Mathieuet et al 1988). Although decreased muscle force may contribute to further minimizing activity level; however increased force of individual muscle force may not help to improve activity level in PD subjects. An increasing strength may not be sufficient to bring about improved walking performance without practice of the action itself, which is necessary for neural adaptation to task and context to be regained (Rutherford 1988). Therefore although strengthening may help to improve force, excitability as well as metabolism of muscles but which may not be sufficient to alter functional status in PD subjects. Only people with very weak individual muscle may be able to alter their functional status to some extent if they practice strengthening exercise. Baatile et al (2000) have demonstrated that individuals with PD who completed an 8 week strengthening program increases perceived functional independence and quality of life. Six male volunteers (average age 72.7) performed *pole striding* exercise three times per week for 37 minutes. Many PD subjects preserve the normal function of individual muscle, and therefore strengthening training may not alter their functional status. Moreover the ability to generalize the result of this study is limited because sample size, and the study did not employ a more rigorous randomized design with a control treatment.

One of the largest difficulties of therapy is generalization of the obtained results to other situations than the therapeutical settings (Hochstenbach and Mulder 1999). During therapy, the world is simplified, protected, predictable hospital environment, while outside patients have to deal with a complex, and ever changing world (Hochstenbach and Mulder 1999). Tulving and Thomson (1973) affirm that the more the final application resembles the practice context, the better the retention performance will be. Therefore it is important PD subjects learn task specific activities in order to change their functional status

The body adapts specifically to the demands imposed upon it, and research over many years has shown that exercise effects tend to be specific to task and context (Rutherford1988). PD subjects experience difficulty to perform functional task due different movement dysfunctions that are resulted from BG dysfunction; moreover synergist action and inhibition of antagonist while performing voluntary activities may be interfered due to muscle rigidity. Therefore one important strategy is to teach functional tasks, which does not the 'organizational structure' of muscles. Since motor skills have a specific organizational structure, they should not arbitrarily be broken for practice (Hochstenbach and Mulder 1999). They further affirm that better and more efficient movement remembering and learning will result from keeping the component of movement sequence that are inter related and dependent on each other together. However Buchner et al (1996) showed that a curvilinear relationship exists between lower limb strength and walking velocity. They pointed out that this relationship reflects a mechanism by which small change in strength may produce relatively large changes in performance in very weak adults, while large changes may have little or no effect in-able bodied adults. Therefore when muscles are beyond a certain task-dependent threshold (a threshold that for most everyday task is well below normal strength values), exercises are required that are task oriented (Carre Shepehard 2004).

Silver and colleagues (2000) have demonstrated in healthy able bodied person an aerobic treadmill training program, three times a week for three months, resulted in increased gait velocity and cadence, and a decreased in the overall time required to perform modified 'get up and go' test. Exercise intensity was individualized and advanced to 40 minutes' training at approximately 60-70% of maximum heart rate reserve. Moreover Teixera-Salmelda et al (1999) assessed subjects general level of physical on the Human Activity Profile, a survay94 activities including transportation, home maintenance, social and physical activities, which are rated according to their required metabolic equivalents. The result indicated that subjects were more able to perform household chores and recreational activities after strengthening and aerobic training. It is intuitive that a relationship should exist between strength and function; however, the nature and of the relationship appears complex and dependent on degree of muscle weakness. Especially in PD subject this relation may even be more complex, given movement difficulties in PD subjects is linked to defective BG function, and despite strength training and improve aerobic capacity PD subjects continue to experience functional difficulties. Morris et al (1994) and Holden et al (2006) suggest that despite the troublesome nature of disorders such as hypokinesia, akinesia, and dyskinesia, people with PD have remarkable capacity to move quickly and with near normal movement size in certain circumstances. For example, when a person with PD performs a simple ballistic task such as pointing to an object or catching a moving ball, the movement size and speed are frequently normal Morris et al (1994). Whereas, when simple movements are integrated into a long or complex action sequence, they are performed slowly and with much more difficulty. Therefore it is evident that aerobic activities or isolated muscle exercises performed in a therapy department may have little or no impact on the difficulties PD subjects encounter within complex home environment. It is observed that many PD subjects preserve normal muscle strength, even in the advance stage of the disease process. Moreover difficulty to perform different functional task in PD subjects has resulted due difficulty to initiate and execute movements, difficulty to perform large amplitude movements, difficulty to perform complicated concurrent movements. Therefore simply strengthening individual muscle or improving aerobic capacity may have insignificant impact on the functional status in PD subjects. In contrast task specific activities may have effective and long-term impact on the functional status in PD subjects. In addition in PD subjects the muscle weakness is attributable to under activity or reduced activity, therefore a strategy to learn to perform functional tasks seems appropriate to hinder development of muscle weakness. Therefore learning functional tasks, which help to overcome difficulties linked to BG degeneration, seem to be appropriate strategy to change functional status of PD subjects.

Carr and Shepherd (2004) suggest that strengthening training that involves repetitive practice of the action being learned can improve strength and endurance if load is progressively increased in some way. However Treiber et al (1998) suggest that transfer of muscle strength into improved functional performance depends on the ability of subject practicing the task. In both strengthening training and skill development repetition is an important aspect of practice (Carr and Shepherd 2004) P 23. Treiber (1998) studied in tennis players, who performed glenohumeral internal and external rotation exercises (incorporating elastic band and hand weight resistance), in standing position, with shoulder in at 90° abduction. The result show a significant increase in force production of the actions practiced, with a transfer into increased speed of serve. Transfer is unlikely to occur, however, unless subject are also practicing the task to be learned (in the above case, the tennis serve), even in some modified context. Paradoxically PD subjects may continue to experience difficulty in performing different tasks, even though the muscle strengthening is achieved in a therapeutic setting, because their task difficulties are linked to basal ganglia dysfunction. It is therefore important that PD subjects learn functional task and then they repeat those tasks during different daily activity. Repetitive practice of the action to be learned can therefore have duel benefits, enabling the patient to practice the action as well as increase muscle strength (Rutherford 1988). Moreover repetition of functional tasks during daily activities can facilitate experience-dependent change in the intact neural circuit of the brain, which in turn will assure long-term change in functional status in PD subjects.

In conclusion it is important that training program uses task-specific activities. Since the BG dysfunction is responsible for the progressive deterioration of functional status, and then development of disability in PD subjects. Moreover task-specific activities allow PD subjects to repeat those tasks during different daily activities, which in turn may have long-term impact on functional status in PD subjects.

X BALANCE FUNCTION IN PARKINSON DISEASE:

Balance is an important function enabling one to perform different activities effectively, and impaired balance reaction may be responsible for the reduce activity level. According to Berg (1989) balance can be viewed as prerequisite to functional activities as it forms the baseline requirement necessary to carry out activities of daily living. Newton (1995) defines standing balance as the ability of individual to maintain or regain the centre of mass over the base of support when faced with altered environmental condition. Berg (1989) further defines balance as maintenance of a position postural adjustment to voluntary movement and in reaction to external disturbances. Moreover Makinnon and Winter (1993) suggests that balance involves the regulation of movement of linked body segments over the supporting joints and over the base of support. Furthermore Carr and Shefered (2003) describe that it is the ability to balance the body mass relative to the base of support that enable us to perform everyday actions effectively and efficiently. Balance is the integrated action of different sensory functions as well as voluntary and involuntary muscle activity. Many Parkinson subjects' reduced activity level may be attributed to the poor balance reaction. However the higher centers for the regulation of balance reaction remains unaffected in Parkinson's disease still there are prevalence of instability and falls among these patients. Moreover Horaket et al (1992) affirms that "pull test" is positive in many Parkinson patients. ("Pull test" consists of sudden a quick and unexpected pulling from backward, provoking balance disturbance of a person. Normal individual react by dorsiflexing their ankles, lifting the arms forward and in some cases flexing forward at the hips and by stepping backward, in case of impaired balance reaction, these reactions are absent or diminished in amplitude). Studies using support-surface perturbation have identified several distinguishing postural abnormalities (Rogers 1996, and Bloem et al 2001):

- Abnormally sized automatic postural responses particularly enlarged "medium latency" stretch responses in lower leg muscles.
- Inability to modulate the response magnitude to different postural demands.
- Delayed initiation or reduced scaling of voluntary postural responses
- Abnormal execution of compensatory stepping movements.

One of the striking features in many PD subjects is falls which may be attributable to impaired balance function, and the fear of falls might force patient to minimize their activity level. Balance impairment and falls are important features of PD. Carr and Shepherd (2004) identify that the likelihood of falling increases in the weak and frail, or in the presence of an impairment affecting the neuromuscular or sensory system, since under these conditions the actions which are normally performed skillfully can no longer be performed effectively. According to the Guideline of Italian neurological society (2003) falls in Parkinson subjects may be due to postural instability and consequent difficulties to readjust in changing postural attitudes or the direction of deambulation, but also freezing, festination dyskinesias or symptomatic orthostatic hypotension. This guideline further suggests that the most frequent causes of acute co-morbidities in Parkinson subjects (about 30% of case) are traumas caused by falls, particularly limb fractures. However Tinitti et al (1988) and Nevitt et al (1989) suggest that falls are equally the main cause of morbidity and mortality in normal elderly subjects and frequently lead to the loss of autonomy and consequent institutionalization, therefore Ammannati et al (1998); Marina et al (1996) suggests that the age and the advance stage of the disease process together represent a particular risk in PD subjects. Therefore fall prevention by improving balance reaction seems to be one of the major strategies in maintaining optimal functional activity level in PD subjects. It seems important to examine the underlying factors that are responsible for the impair balance function in PD. These factors include neurotransmitter disturbance, which is attributable to basal ganglia degeneration, postural change, and muscle dysfunction (rigidity, akinesia, weakness and shortening of muscles). The following discussion tries to examine these underlying factors so that appropriate measures can be taken to improve balance function in PD.

X 1. Neurotransmitter disturbance and balance function in PD:

A neurotransmitter disturbance associated with basal ganglia degeneration contributes to impair balance function in Parkinson patients. Elble (1998) describes that reason why balance is disrupted is unclear, although it appears to be associated with neurotransmitter disturbances in the output projections from the internal globus palladus to the midbrain and brain-stem regions involved in maintaining upright stance and extensor muscle activity. Advanced stage of the disease processes the postural change, muscle weakness, and muscle shortening may further aggravation impaired balance function, whereas these problems are preventable if adequate measures are taken.

X2 Posture change and balance impairment in PD:

Berg (1989) describes that in quite standing, the centre of mass situated in the midline and slightly anterior of the sacral region. Any movement usually accompanied or proceeded by a counterbalancing of another body segment so that the body's centre of gravity remains over the centre of base of support. In Parkinson disease a generalised flexion posture may displace the centre of mass and consequently accentuate the instability of the patient. Wissenborn. (1993) postulates that the biomechanical impairments related to Parkinson patients' poor posture might well contribute to the desequilibrium and instability. According to Wyke (1979) the abnormalities in the cervical spine reduce the efficiency of postural control and contribute to the disorders of posture and gait. Therefore in Parkinson disease flexion deformity of cervical and thoraco-lumbar spine may displace body's centre of gravity away from the centre of mass, which may be responsible for the instability and falls.

X3 Muscle function and balance control in PD:

Postural readjustment: Voluntary and involuntary muscle function play an important role in balance control and the prevention of falls. Rigidity of muscle and different factors responsible for the akinetic syndrome may in turn be responsible for the falls. This is often mainly due to difficulty to readjust in case of sudden postural change. Massion (1992) affirms that the rigidity does not allow the locomotor organs to readapt effectively in case change of position, and there may be imperfect muscle response due to akinesia. According to Bleton and Stevenin (1988) the Parkinson patients have impaired balance reaction not because of impairment of the higher centre for balance regulation but due to difficulty in automatic postural readjustment.

Muscle shortening: Tendoachilis (triceps sural) shortening may be responsible for the altered alignment of the body resulting in a poor stability. Carr and Shefered (2003) describe that contracture and stiffness of muscles, particularly soleus, may restrict the ability to balance and may be cause of fall in elderly individuals. They further suggest that short cuff muscles interfere with hip extension in standing and walking and a short soleus interfere with initial foot placement backward and standing up. In Parkinson subjects often these two muscles may be shorten progressively due to inactivity or reduced activity level, resulting in postural instability and falls.

Muscle weakness: Weakness of lower limb muscle may be responsible for the postural instability and falls. Fiatarone et al (1990), Johanosson and Jarnlo (1991) have demonstrated that lower limb strengthening exercise programme can have positive effect in balance and gait performances. Reduced activity level in PD may be responsible for the weakness of lower limb muscles leading to impaired balance function. It is evident postural instability and falls in Parkinson disease are partly due to akinesia of movement and rigidity of muscles, but the major factors that contribute to the impaired balance are change of postural alignment of the body, muscle shortening and muscle weakness. The later causes are often results from reduced activity level, and may be prevented by maintaining improved activity level.

Conclusion:

It can be concluded that although the higher centre for the balance reaction remains intact, still impaired balance function leading to falls are prevalent in Parkinson subjects. Several factors are indeed responsible for the poor balance function and falls in PD, they include imbalance of the neurotransmitter, difficulty to carry out a postural readjustment in case of sudden change of posture due to the muscle rigidity and different underlying factors of akinesia; muscle shortening, which may deviate the line of gravity away from the centre of mass of the body thus aggravate instability, and finally weakness muscles of the lower limbs may be responsible for the fall and balance impairment. Therefore it seems prerequisite to strengthening balance function to improve functional activity level.

Ellis et al (2005) affirm that people with PD have difficulty with task such as walking, rising from chair, and moving in bed, and this decrease in functional status often results in a loss of independence and a decline in quality of life (QOL). According to Morris (2000) movement disorders are hallmark of PD and can severely compromise an individual's ability to perform well-learned motor skills such as walking, turning around, transferring in and out of bed (Morris 2000).

It is described earlier that the BG dysfunction results in an impairment of selective perceiving and responding of movement during different functional tasks,

However as PD is a degenerative disease as the degeneration progresses there are less and less dopaminergic neurones left to carry out the function of the nigrostiatal system. Moreover not only nigrostraital system but also in the advance state of the disease the whole BG may be subjected to a degenerative change, in which case even the administration of dopamine may not enhance its function. Therefore often a honey-moon period is observed in PD subject when the efficacy of dopamine is at its maximum, after which the effectiveness of dopamine becomes non-significant.

IX

Cognitive Impairments in PD Subjects and their Repercussion on Functional Activity Level

Studies of patients with Parkinson's disease suggest that the characteristic motor symptoms are frequently accompanied by impairments in cognitive function (Lewis et al 2003). Côté and Crutcher (1991) affirm that patients with Parkinson's disease have disturbances of affective as well as cognitive function. Given that the basal ganglia have extensive connection with the different regions of the brain, which may also explain that an impaired neurotransmitter metabolism in BG and their connection may result in a cognitive dysfunction.

According to the guideline for the treatment of Italian Neurological society about 20% Parkinsonian patients experience a specific cognitive impairment like memory, attention, and alteration of executive function. One-fifth of urgent admissions to neurological departments are due to acute cognitive-behavioural deficiencies (Sanchez-Ramoset et al 1996). Brown and Marsden (1986) and DellaSalla et al (1996) have reported the discrete impairment of visuospatial abilities; Stern et al (1987); Raskin et al (1989) have reported the impairment of frontal function; and Owen et al (1998) have established impairment of memory function. Uekermann et al (2004) state that examination of cognitive function often reveals mild to moderate deficits, including visuospatial impairment, attention set-sifting difficulties, working memory impairment and poor executive function. Different cognitive dysfunction can not only have interfering effect in retrieving organised motor activities during functional tasks but also the process of experience-dependent changes in the intact neural circuits may not be facilitated in PD subjects, which hinder the brain's ability to readjust with the impaired BG function. Therefore it is often observed an accelerated disabling process in PD subjects with severe cognitive dysfunction.

The following discussion integrates clinical research findings on the role of BG in mediating cognitive function. Given that attention and executive dysfunction are two common dysfunctions in PD therefore the discussion integrate the available clinical and research findings to provide therapists with more insight on the interaction of these two cognitive deficits in PD subjects.

XI1 Role of basal ganglia in the regulation of cognitive function:

The functions of basal ganglia are long been recognised as to be involved in generation of different motor functions; however the detailed investigation of anatomy and physiology of basal ganglia makes it evident that they are also responsible for other functions like cognitive and emotional function. A wide range of motor and non motor behaviours have been correlated with activity in individual basal ganglia neurons in experimental animals and with the metabolic activity in the basal ganglia as seen by the imaging studies in humans (Kandel et al 2000). The functional anatomy of the basal ganglia may be defined in terms of five functional loops, which include motor, occulomotor, dorsolateral, prefrontal, lateral orbitofrontl, and anterior cingulated and they constitute feed-forward and feed-back pathways between basal ganglia themselves and between the basal ganglia and other cortical structures (Alexander et al 1986). These functional loops are not only responsible for the generation motor function but also regulate different cognitive and behaviour function. For example disruption of motor and oculomotor loops may result in pure motor deficit; dorsolateral and lateral orbitomedial prefrontal loops may produce cognitive deficit, or disruption of limbic loop result in emotional deficits (Afifi 1993). Moreover disturbances in of the dopaminergic system are thought to play a role in the development of frontal executive impairment (Godefroy 2003). Altered striatal outflow to the frontal cortex in PD suggests that striatal structures mediate executive functioning (Elliott 2003). PD-related changes are describes in prefrontal regions (Fuster 1996) participating in "cognitive" basal ganglia-thalamocortical circuits (Marie and Defer 2003). Sammer et al (2006) suggest that orbitofrontal and dorsolateral circuits different aspect of executive functioning. The orbitofrontal circuit is involved in inhibitory control (Weintraub et al 2005), for instant in the context of task processing with in an interfering environment (Dujardin et al 1999), or in the inhibition of ineffective behavioural strategies (Bokura et al 2004, Brand et al 2004). Moreover dorso lateral activation can frequently be found in the working memory task, for instance in the planning and sequencing task (Weintraub et al 2005). Therefore Sammer et al (2006) summarised that selective cognitive impairment in PD is associated with decrements in working memory that require executive processing, including frontal lobe dysfunction. The authors further affirm that each of these five basal ganglia-thalamocortical circuits appear to receive input from several but functionally related cortical areas, traverse specific portions of the basal ganglia and thalamus, and then project back upon the same cortical areas providing input to the circuit, thus forming partially closed loops. The hippocampus and the caudate nucleus are essential structures for the elimination of responses to irrelevant stimuli, enabling organism to behave in a strictly selective manner; and a lesion of these structures is the source of the breakdown of selective behaviour, which in fact more a disturbance of selective attention than a defect of memory. In fact basal ganglia function like a "clearing house" that accumulates sample of ongoing cortical activity and on competitive basis, can facilitate any one and suppress others, that they have important role in selective responding (Denny-Brown and Yanagisawa 1976). This selection of stimuli and prioritising seems essential during simultaneous movement while performing functional activities, which in fact enables one to switch from one movement to another without much difficulty. Similar problem arises during selection and prorating activities of daily living. Therefore it is evident that the basal ganglia play important role in regulation of some cognitive functions, and its dysfunction may impair cognitive function.

XI3 Attention dysfunction in PD:

Zomeren and Brower (1994) define attention as a cognitive state characterised by a selective bias for processing certain internal and external stimuli. Attention function may be impaired in Parkinson subjects. The finding on animal study suggests that the basal ganglia play a role in corticosubcortico control loops that modulate the state of preparation of cortex (Marsden 1982). Moreover the basal ganglia and limbic system particularly the afferent part of basal ganglia, which consists of caudate nucleus and putamen are probably involved in the selective component of attention (Van Zomeren and Brouwer 1994). A neurotransmitter dysfunction within the basal ganglia may result in an impairment of attention function. The attention is essential not only for the generation of organised motor activities but also in case of difficulty to organised motor activities conscious attention help overcome difficulty. Moreover relearning of motor activities, generating bilateral alternative movements, facilitating experience-dependent change in the intact neural circuits the attention function has a crucial role. The following discussion integrate clinical research findings to provide therapists with some insights on the impaired attention in PD subjects, and some of the strategies to minimise the effects of attention dysfunction.

XI5 the effects of impaired attention in Parkinson subjects:

Many PD subjects have to reliant on attention while performing functional activities. Morris et al (1998) and Behrman et al (1998) suggest that PD subjects who are cognitively intact simply focusing attention on the critical aspect of movement that need to be controlled can be sufficient to activate with near-normal speed and size. Because the cortical regions remain unaffected by the disease in the early stages, the person appears to be able to use "online" frontal-lobe cognitive strategy to compensate for the BG insufficiency (Morris 2000). Moreover the failure to generate organised kinematic motor activities, PD subject has to learn to disintegrate the complex motor activities into several simple tasks and then pay attention to each task separately to produce a purposeful task.

XI4 Role of attention in re-learning of motor activities:

Learning of motor strategies to overcoming the movement difficulties resulted from PD is essential and attention disorder may have adverse consequence on this relearning process. Hochtenbach and Mulder (1999) state that attention forms not only a prerequisite for almost all human actions and is of crucial importance for effective human behaviour and survival, it also plays a major role in the (re) acquisition of skills. According to Theeuwis (1992) attention is necessary for the correct perception of conjunctions, although unattended features are conjoined prior to conscious perception. The top-down processing of unattended features is capable of utilizing past experience and contextual information. Moreover difficulty to generate organised kinematic motor activities, many PD subject have to be reliant on attention function to overcome movement difficulty. Attention system has important role in registering, and processing of all information received by the individual. (Hochchstenbach and Mulder (1999) suggest that attention processes guide the selective pick-up of information; whereas memory processes are responsible for the storage of this information. A relevant task is more easily attended than irrelevant tasks. Function tasks constitute relevant stimulation for the brain and only the relevant stimulation may be picked up by the attention system. In contrast the unattended stimulation may be lost before it reaches to the memory process. The functional tasks not only constitute the relevant information for the memory but also repeating those tasks during daily activities open up the opportunity to rehearse them. In this context learning of isolated movements and group gymnastic in a therapy department though effective for the general well being, they constitute irrelevant information may not be attended by the brain and unable to reach short-term or log term memory. Mak and Hui-Chan (2008) found that audiovisual cued sit-to-stand training produced better sit-to-stand initiation and execution than those who performed isolated exercise. The selective attention to audiovisual cues have enhanced explicit learning leading to declarative knowledge of the movement sequence (Kelly et al 2004), then with repeated sit-to-stand practice these declarative knowledge have translated into procedural knowledge (Pasual-Leone 1993). Moreover

Mak and Hui-Chan (2008) further suggest that the task-specific training strategy with audiovisual cues could have produced plastic changes in the brain of PD subjects than those of exercise training alone. Therefore PD subjects with impaired attention function may experience difficulty to learn the novel movement strategy to cope with movement dysfunction resulted from BG dysfunction.

XI6 Role of attention in generating bilateral alternative movements in Parkinson subjects:

One of the major difficulties that Parkinson subjects encounter is the difficulty to generate bilateral alternative movements. The spatial attention system generates alternative bilateral activation and inhibition during different functional tasks (Robetson 1999). Furthermore two mutually facilitation process, that is arousal/sustained-attention system of the brain in one hand, and spatial-attention system on the other hand responsible for the producing bilateral alternative movements (Robertson 1999). Therefore impaired attention to a certain extent is responsible the difficulty to generate bilateral alternative movements during walking and turning. However, further research is required to establish the relationship between impaired bilateral and alternative movements, and attention disorder in Parkinson subjects.

XI7 Repercussion of attention disorder in neural reorganisation:

The most damaging effect of impair attention system seems to be failure to facilitate experience-dependent change in the intact neural circuits, because these types of changes largely depend on the intact attention system. Experience-dependent change in the intact neural circuits depends on attention being paid by the recipient to the stimulation responsible for such change (Recanzone et al 1993). Given that PD subject with impaired attention are not able to facilitate experience-dependent change in the intact neural circuits, they might experience difficulty to relearn novel movement strategies to cope with functional difficulties. Furthermore rehabilitation of attention is an important goal itself as an intervening step in rehabilitation of other types of cognitive, motor and perceptual function, given that attention is a key element of experience-dependent change Robertson (1999).

XI 8 Possible strategy minimise the effects of attention dysfunction in PD:

One important consideration is that the attention system has four distinct parts and it may be possible that all four aspects are not be impaired in PD; it is therefore important to identify the aspect of attention that are intact. Although there is considerable disagreements regarding several attention models in term of capacity, filter characteristics, time-sharing abilities, control mechanisms, multiple or unitary resources a distinction on several aspect of attention are made; like selective attention, focused attention, divided attention, and sustained attention (van Zomeren and Brower 1994). Selective attention can be seen as a perceptual filtering out of all one single input source on the basis of task and context variables and on the physical characteristic of the input source(s), and selective attention essential to perform task accurately especially if it requires precision, using conscious awareness (Hochtenbach and Mulder 1999). Selective attention seems important to perform many activities, especially when PD subjects can no longer relay on spontaneous activities of program controlled system, the selective attention may help to reduce the delay in initiation and execution of movements. Focused attention enables one to direct the attention to the main aspect of a task without being distracted irrelevant stimuli (Hochtenbach and Mulder 1999). The ability to pick up information from an environment in such a way, that enables one to follow a particular flow of information while ignoring potential distracters with a remarkable ease (e.g. 'coctail party effect'), and this is identified as focused attention (Hochstenbach and Mulder 1999). Moreover focused attention plays important role in generating purposeful, effective movement, while ignore undesired movements during functional activities.

Focused attention is important in selecting appropriate movement and not disturbed by previously constructed movements. One strategy to overcome the task difficulties is to disintegrate the complicated movements with in a task in to several simple movements and then focus attention in each aspect of the movement. Focusing attention in each aspect of movement can eventually facilitate experience dependent change in the intact neural circuit and the new experience can eventually transform into knowledge.

Divided attention seems to reflect one's capacity to shift between several inputs sources or tasks and to do two or more things simultaneously, where as sustain attention the ability to concentrate on a given task over long generally unbroken periods of time without a substantial decline or large fluctuation in the performance (Hochtenbach and Mulder 1999). Therefore it is essential to identify the aspect of attention that is intact, and then use the intact aspect to overcome movement difficulty.

In conclusion attention has important role in the generation of kinematic organised motor activities; it has a crucial role in motor relearning process; moreover experience dependent in the brain is dependent on attention being paid by the recipient to the stimulation responsible for such change. However attention function has four distinct parts and it is worthwhile to identify the aspect of attention remains intact, which might help PD subject to compensate the attention dysfunction.

In conclusion

- attention has important role in the generation of kinematic organised motor activities;
- it has a crucial role in motor learning process;
- moreover experience-dependent in the brain is dependent on attention being paid by the recipient to the stimulation responsible for such change.

However attention function has four distinct parts and it is worthwhile to identify the aspect of attention remains intact, which might help PD subject to compensate the attention dysfunction.

XI 8 Impaired of executive function in PD:

The executive function is defined as those capacities that enable a person to engage successfully in independent, purposive, self-serving behaviour no matter how well they can see and hear, walk and talk and perform tests (Lezak 1995). According to Smith and Jonides (1999) the term 'executive functions' refers to a whole range of adaptive abilities such as creative and abstract thought, introspection, forming plan, based on recollections of past experiences. These abilities play a crucial part in complex social and domestic behaviour, help to suppress improper actions and focus on purposeful information. The translation of an intention or plan into productive, self-serving activity requires the actor to initiate, maintain, switch, and stop sequences of complex behaviour in an orderly and integrated manner and disturbances in the programming of activity can thwart the carrying out of reasonable plans regardless of motivation, knowledge, or capacity to perform the activity (Lezak 1995). It can be extremely difficult for the people with executive dysfunction to control their own lives, and they almost fully dependent on external structures, routine, and other people, with little room for flexibility (Hochestbach and Mulder 1999). They further affirm that the extent of dependency varies with the seriousness of the dysexecutive syndrome and with the presence of other cognitive and emotional disorders.

XI 9 The basal ganglia and impaired executive function:

The pattern of cognitive impairment seen in the early stages of PD resembles that produced by frontal lobe damage and includes deficits of executive functions, such as planning and working-memory (Lee et al 1998; and Taylor et al 1986). Moreover some Parkinson subjects display diminished conceptual flexibility and impaired spontaneity (Lezak 1995). Functional neuroimaging studies suggest that executive dysfunction in PD is related to both disruption of in the nigrostraital (Owen et al 1998; Dagher et al 2001) mesocortical (Cools et al 2002; Mattay et al 2002) pathways. However in the early stage of the disease process the mesocortical projection is far less severely affected than the nigrostraital dopamine system (Agid et al 1987). Study with event-related functional magnetic resonance brain imaging (fMRI) demonstrate that a subgroup of PD patients with a selective executive deficit exhibit significant under activation in the striatum as well as in the frontal cortex during performance of a working-memory task, compared to patients with no significant executive memory impairments (Lewis et al 2003). Moreover bilateral caudate under activity in the executively impaired subgroup patients is observed compare to those patients with no impairment, therefore it may be assumed that these structures may play a more specific role in cognitive function (Rinne et al 1989). This is equally observed in animal lesion experiments, which suggests that the caudate nuclei may play specific role in cognition (Divac et al 1967). Most probably degeneration or under activity of caudate nucleus may responsible for the depletion of dopamine resulting in impaired cognitive function, especially executive function.

XI 10 Role of dopamine on executive function:

Lack of dopamine seems to be responsible for the impaired executive function. Dopamine deficit has been suggested to be extremely sensitive to impairment of executive function effect (Lange et al 1992). Lewis et al (2003) suggest that the cognitive deficit in PD may reflect nigrostriaital dopaminergic depletion and its disruptive influence on the functioning of frontostraital territory. Moreover a correlation between loss of dopamirgic neurons at the dorsomedial projection of the nigro-straital tract and the degree of dementia observed in PD subjects (Rinne et al 1989). The imaging finding study conducted by Lewis et al (2003) has demonstrated that a subgroup of PD subjects with selective executive deficit exhibit significant under activation in the striatum as well as frontal cortex during performance of working memory task, compare to patient with no significant executive impairments. However this under activation in the executively impaired subgroup of PD subjects is not a global effect, because there are no differences between patient subgroups in the posterior association cortices, which are also known to play a role in working memory (Owen et al 1998b). Therefore, it is more likely that that dopaminergic depletion and its disruptive influence on the functioning of frontostraital circuitry can be responsible for the dysexecutive syndrome.

XI11 Repercussion of executive function on functional activity level in Parkinson subjects:

Parkinson subjects with disorder in executive function would be unable to plan and then take necessary actions in performing activities of daily living, therefore they may not be able to initiate and execute activities of daily living. Lezak (1982) argued that for the performance of goal-directed behaviour four components are important, they are :

- (1) one has to formulate a goal or an intention,
- (2) one has to plan the different steps needed to achieve the goal,
- (3) one has to translate the plan into purposeful action, which requires the ability to initiate maintain, switch, and stop ongoing behaviour, and
- (4) one has to perform effectively, which requires the ability to make use of the response-produced feedback.

In a dysexecutive syndrome one or several aspects of those goal directed behaviour may be impaired. Moreover the disorders do not only exist at the level of actions, but also at the level of thinking, which is reflected in the problem these patients may have in arranging and integrating their thoughts and experiences (Hochstenbach and Mulder 1999). Despite the fact that the motor activities remain intact still patients with executive dysfunction may dependent on other people for the activities of daily living, and it seems that this passive way of living may have negative impact on the mechanism of neural recovery.

Although programming functions are necessary for the successful performance of non-routine tasks; but are not needed when the action sequence is routine (Shallice 1982). Therefore over learned familiar, routine tasks and automatic behaviour can be expected to be much less vulnerable to brain damage than are non-routine or novel activities (Lezak 1995). Probably for this reason many Parkinson subjects perform their activities of daily living in an obsessively ritual way; that is they perform same function in the same time every day. This type of rigid routine living style is one of the compensatory strategies to cope with dysexecutive syndrome. Although akinesia and muscle rigidity are often responsible for the limited activity level and ritual way of leading the activities of daily living, however it seems that impaired executive function is also responsible for this rigid living style in number of PD subjects. The most damaging effect of impaired executive function, where PD subjects are dependent on other people for the every task of daily living, and they may unlikely to foster changes like functional reorganisation or experience-dependent change in the neural circuits of the brain.

X12 Research on executive function in PD subjects:

Sammer et al (2006) conducted a research study on 26 PD subjects. The aim of the study was to analyse the effect of cognitive treatment on cognitive performance. The half of the subjects participated in a cognitive training regimen, while other half only received standard treatment. The outcome showed improved performance of the group with cognitive treatment in two executive tasks after the training period, while no improvement was seen in the standard-treatment group.

The results indicate that specific training is required improvement of executive functions, while general rehabilitation is not sufficient. Therefore they recommended that PD subject might benefit from short-term cognitive executive function training program that is tailored to individual patient's need. However this research had not explored the repercussion of improved executive function on functional activity level in PD subjects.

Conclusion:

Neurotransmitter metabolism dysfunction in the BG may impair attention function, which is an important cognitive function. Basal ganglia mainly regulate the selective attention, which enables one to prioritise muscle activities in complex functional task. The selective attention not only mediate in selecting and prioritising muscle function but also in complex social or domestic events the selective attention interact in selecting and prioritising process. Attention impairment can severely hinder peoples' relearning abilities. It may aggravate the disabling process given that many PD subjects may relay on attention to compensate movement disorder. In addition attention system has a privileged role in fostering experience-dependent change in the intact neural circuits; therefore, its impairment may interfere in neural remodelling and thus Parkinson subject may not be able effectively counteract different movement dysfunctions.

Basal ganglia degeneration may also be responsible for the impaired executive function. The executive function is defined as those capacities that enable a person to engage successfully in independent, purposive, self-serving behaviour no matter how well they can see and hear, walk and talk and perform tests (Lezak 1995). It is equally observed that there is a correlation between reduce dopamine and dysexecutive syndrome. PD subjects with selective executive deficit exhibit significant under activation in the striatum as well as frontal cortex during performance of working memory task. Impaired executive function may severely reduce activity level in Parkinson subjects. It seems important to identify the cognitive impairments in PD and adapt physiotherapy treatment according to the impaired cognitive function.

Summary of cognitive dysfunction in PD subjects:

> 6. Basal ganglia regulate a wide range of cognitive function
> 7. A large majority of people with Parkinson's disease have different degrees of cognitive impairment, the common impairment include attention and executive dysfunction
>
> The repercussion of impair attention function can include:
> 8. The use of conscious attention can help PD subject to activate movements with near-normal speed and size.
> 9. Impaired attention can severely hinder relearning of movement strategy to cope with movement difficulties resulted from PD;
> 10. bilateral alternative movements pattern may be impaired given attention function mediate the generation of bilateral alternative movement
> 11. Attention dysfunction can have hindering effect on experience-dependent change in the intact neural circuits of the brain

> The repercussion of impaired executive function include:
> 12. The activity level of Parkinson subjects may severely reduce in PD subjects with executive dysfunction.
> 13. Parkinson subjects with dysexecutive syndrome may be dependent on other people for the activities of daily living; the disability will depend on the severity of dysexecutive syndrome, and the presence of other cognitive dysfunction.

X

Possibility to Foster Neural Changes in Parkinson Subjects in Order to Assure Long Term Functional Improvement

Introduction: New brain imaging techniques are making it clear that the neural system is continuously remodelling throughout the life by experience and learning in response to activities and behaviour (Jankins et al 1990; Johansson 2000; Nudo et al 2001). However Parkinson disease is degenerative disease and there is no data available suggesting the extent of neural changes that can be facilitated in Parkinson subjects. One important aspect of Parkinson disease is that wide areas of motor controlling system remain intact, therefore it may be predicted that a functional and structural change on those areas may be facilitated by providing 'planned experience' or appropriate therapy. Rehabilitation – the provision of planned experience to foster brain changes leading to improved daily life functioning – can now therefore turn its sights to the ambitious goal of directly altering neural circuitry through appropriate planned experience (Robertson 1999).

The following discussion reviews briefly the possible atrophy and degeneration of basal ganglia link to stress deprivation and anti Parkinson drug; the different literature on experience-dependent change and functional reorganisation in human and in animal and the possibility to foster those changes on PD subjects' brain.

XII 1Task-specific training to slow degeneration of dopamine producing cells and facilitate neuroprotection:

Evidences from animal model suggest that pharmacotherapies, learning and exercise may have neuroprotctive influence in neurological disorders (Woodlee and Schallert 2004; Spires and Hannan2005). Woodlee and Schallert (2004) found that the onset of abnormal movements to be prevented or delayed when parkinsonian rats exposed to MPTP (1-methyl-4-phenyl-1,2,3,6-tetrahydropyridine) were trained in an enriched environment. Similarly, rat models of Huntington disease have shown that locomotor training using a treadmill within an enriched environment delays the progression of gait disorders (Spires and Hannan2005). Fisher et al (2002) demonstrated that in medication induced PD rats, treadmill walking for 30 days resulted in walking speed being recovered to the level of nonlesioned animals, along with increased synaptic occupancy of dopamine receptors in the brain. Moreover according to Tillerson (2002) goal directed, learning-based training can contribute to enriched function in people with neurodegenerative conditions. If animal finding could be generalised in human, task-specific training could induce plastic change in the brain of human PD (Mak and Hui-Chan 2008). Moreover Mak and Hui-Chan (2008) found that task-specific training strategy with audiovisual (AV) cues have produced more plastic changes in the brain than of exercise alone, leading to carry-over improvement to noncued environment and to at least 2 weeks after training ended. However people with impaired cognitive function may not be able to facilitate these types of plastic changes, given cognitive function especially attention function plays an important role in learning process and eventual facilitation of experience-dependent change in the intact neural circuits in the brain.

Fisher et al (2008) studied thirty people with PD, within 3 years of diagnosis with Hoehn and Yahr stage 1or 2. The objective of the study is to investigate the effects of high-intensity exercise on functional performance in people with PD relative to exercise at low and no intensity, and to determine whether improved performance is accompanied by alteration in corticomotor excitability as measured through transcranial magnetic stimulation (TMS). The result showed that a small improvement in total and motor Unified Parkinson Disease Rating Scale (UPRS) in all groups. High-intensity group subjects showed post-exercise increases in gait speed, step and stride length, and hip and ankle joint excursion during self-selected and fast and improved weight distribution during sit-to-stand tasks. However the improvements in gait and sit-to-stand measures were not consistently observed in low and zero-intensity groups. Moreover the high-intensity group showed lengthening in cortical silent period. Therefore the authors concluded from this study that the dose-depended benefits of exercise and high-intensity exercise can normalise corticomotor excitability in early Parkinson disease.

Under-activity or reduced activity may deprive different areas of basal ganglia and their connection of adequate stimulation enhancing their degenerative process in a similar way the musculo-skeletal system undergo degenerative changes as a result of stress deprivation. Research on primate has demonstrated that the neurons at the brain that are deprived of normal stress may be atrophied. For example research by Nudo et al (1996) on squirrel monkey showed that following a lesion to a small part of motor cortex, hand-movement representations adjacent to the area of infarct that were spared from direct injury underwent further loss of hand cortical territory in the absence of intensive training. Moreover Lewis et al (2003) used even related functional magnetic resonance imaging (fMIR) on people with executive dysfunction and demonstrated that there was specific under-activity in the striatum as well as in the frontal cortex during performance of working-memory task compare to group with no significant executive impairments. It is therefore evident that reduced functional activity may be responsible for the under activity of BG neurons; and this under activity of neurons may be responsible for their atrophy and further degeneration. In contraire early treatment targeting up-regulating of dopamine producing neurons might slow the progression of the PD (Woodlee et al 2004). Therefore optimising activity level seems to have neuroprotective influence, which may contribute to slowing the disabling process in PD subjects. However most researches on neuroprotective influence are done on animal; to date there are no longitudinal studies confirming that meticulous commitment to learning in patient diagnosed with PD would actually sow down the progression of the disease (Morris 2006). Therefore the author suggests that physiotherapists should collaborate with basic science researchers to improve our understanding of how movement strategies and exercise can be maximally protective.

XII 2 Experience-dependent change:

Research carried out by Eriksson et al (1998) and Gould et al (1999) suggest that in the hippocampus in adult human brain the new cells can be produced. Similarly Gould et al (1997), Kempermann, et al (1997) and Cameron (1993) have demonstrated from stereological analyses that several thousand hipcamppal cells produced each day in adult animals, the majority of which differentiate into granulate neurones. Kaplan et al (1984) reported after experiment on rodent the presence of synapses on cell bodies and dendrites of 3H-thymidine-leveled cells in the dentate gyrus. Stanfield and Trice (1988) found evidence of new cells in extending axons in the dentate gyrus of adult rats. Moreover Gould et al (1999) suggest that if granule neurons produced in adulthood is necessary for hipocampal function in certain types of learning and memory, then regulatory factors that diminish the production of new neurons should be associated with impaired learning while those that enhance the production of new neurones should improve learning. There are ample evidences that new cells are produced in human brain however their retention depends on the types of stimulations people are subjected to.

Moreover study conducted by Cao et al (2002) has demonstrated that lesion-induced cell loss facilitate cell proliferative activities that is loss of cells in one area of the brain facilitate cell proliferation on the other areas, possibly to facilitate the compensation of functional losses. Cao et al (2002) conclude from their research that adult brain of mammals and birds are not generally endowed with mechanisms of cell repair. They however, suggest that lesion and/or lesion-induced cell loss facilitate cell proliferative activity in subventricular zone, concurrently induced morphological changes which may provide a favourable environment for local neuron recruitment. Moreover research carried out by Recanzone et al (1993) has demonstrated that following brain damage, the adult brain can show large experience-dependent change in the intact neural circuits, including dendritic and axonal sprouting. Increase in synaptic efficacy in the existing neural circuits in the form of long-term potential and formation of new synapses may be essential for the earlier stage of motor learning (Asanuma and Keller1991). These evidences may suggest that degeneration of subsentia niagra may facilitate proliferation of new neurons as well as axonal and dendritic sprouting on the other areas of the brain. However retention of newly proliferated cells including axonal and dendritic sprouting largely depends on different activities performed; in contrast inactivity may favour their disintegration. This is affirmed by Kempermann et al (1998) and they suggest that the process of neurognesis (production of nerve cells) is partly experience-dependent. That is proliferation and the retention of new cells and different axonal and dendritic sprouting depends on the stimulations received by the recipient. Kempermann et al (1998) have demonstrated that more hippocampal granule neurons are maintained in mice living in 'enriched environment' conditions compared to laboratory cage control. Praag.et al (1999) demonstrate running; and Gould et al (1999) demonstrate specific learning tasks promote neurogenesis and neural survival in the adult mouse hippocampus.

However Gould et al (1999) argue that the extent to which the increase in the number of surviving granule cells following environmental enrichment directly contribute to improved hippocampal function remains unknown.

Moreover there is emerging evidence in animal models that pharmacotherapy, learning, and exercise may have a neuroprotective influence in neurological disorders. Woodlee and Schallert (2004) found that the onset of abnormal movements to be prevented or delayed when parkinsonien rats exposed to MPTP (1-methyl-4-phenyl-1,2,3,6-tetrahydropyridine) were trained in an enriched environment. Similarly Rat models on Huntinton disease have shown that locomotor training using a treadmill within enriched environment delays the progression of gait disorders Spiers et al (2005). However more research is required to validate if the progression of disease process can be delayed if PD subjects live in enriched environment with repeated training and practice.

It can be assumed that the proliferation and retention of new brain cells are facilitated in people or animal living in an enriched environment compared to those living in a deprived environment. These evidences might be used to reason that in PD the new brain cells are produced, that there are lesion-induced cell proliferative activities, and that there is propagation of axonal and dendritic sprouting in the intact neural circuits. Finally learning to perform function tasks using cortically controlled movements and then repeat those tasks may facilitate structural and functional changes in the intact motor neural circuits. Moreover neural adaptation raises the possibility that goal directed, learning-based training can contribute to enhanced function in people with neurodegenerative conditions (Tillerson et al 2002) However there is paucity of research-based evidence regarding the possibility neural changes and enhance functional activity level in PD subjects. It is therefore important to identify the therapeutic activities that constitute the goal-directed, learning-based training for PD subjects for fostering changes in the intact areas of the brain. However Recanzone et al (1993) describe that experience-dependent plastic reorganisation depends on attention being paid by the recipient to the stimulation for such changes, and according to Robertson et al (1997) the attentional systems of the brain might have a privileged role in the recovery of function after brain damage. Whereas many Parkinson subjects may have attention disorder and therefore, it might be difficult to foster these types of changes. Similarly other cognitive dysfunctions like impaired executive function or memory dysfunction may have hindering effect on the proliferation of brain cells as well as dendritic and axonal sprouting. In other word people with cognitive dysfunction may be considered as living in a deprived environment. Moreover, little is known about the parameters such as timing, duration, and the frequency of different stimulations to obtain this type of experience-dependent change (Robertson 1999). One theory put forward by Carre and Shepherd (2004) suggests that the changes in the brain cells associated with skill development can be provoked by active, repetitive training and practice, and by the continued practice of the activity. In Parkinson subjects it is essential to repeat different skills and then integrate those skills in activities of daily living. It is assumed repeated of activities during different functional task (using an alternative strategy) may help to facilitate an experience-dependent change at the level of intact neurons of the motor cortex in PD. Conversely inactivity and lack of stimulation may deprive the intact areas of brain to facilitate functional reorganisation that is a non-challenging environment may hinder this process and thus people may not be able to improve their activity level. Similarly bout exercise programme in PT department may have little impact on neural change in PD subjects.

Therefore it can be concluded that different stimulations may foster experience-dependent change, which include proliferation of new neurons, and axonal and dendritic sprouting in normal subjects and in animals. These changes are experience-dependent that is animals in enriched environment keep on proliferating axonal and dendritic spouting; whereas animals in impoverished environment are deprived of this process. Animal models on Parkinson's disease Woodlee and Schallert(2004) and Huntigton disease as well as healthy animal have demonstrated the neural changes with training Spires et al (2005). Moreover human models there is specific under-activity in the striatum as well as in the frontal cortex during performance of working-memory task compare to group with no significant executive impairments Lewis et al (2003). However, further research is needed to elucidate in what extent these types of changes may be facilitate in PD as well as identify the type of stimulations that may facilitate these changes.

XII 3Functional reorganisation:

Another theory regarding neural recovery is a possible 'functional reorganisation' in the intact neural circuits- the compensatory reorganisation of unaffected brain circuits in order to achieved the impaired functional goals in a different way (Lauria 1963; Lauria et al 1975). Modern cortical mapping techniques in both non-human and human subject indicate that the functional organisation of the primary motor cortex is much more complex than was traditionally described (Carr and Shepherd 2004). Moreover the complex organisation has extensive overlapping of muscle representation within the motor map, with individual muscle and joint representations re-represented within the motor map, individual corticospinal neurons diverging to multiple motoneuron pools, and horizontal fibres interconnecting distributed representations and this complex organisation may provide the foundation for functional plasticity in the motor cortex (Nudo et al 2001). Elbert et al (1995) observed that right-handed string players show an increased cortical representation (map) of flexor and extensor muscles. It is observed that the sensorimotor cortical representation of the reading finger is expanded in blind Braille readers (Pascal-Leone and Torres 1993) and fluctuates according to the extent of reading activities (Pascal-Leone et al 1995). These types of cortical representations (map) remain enlarged with regular practice Elbart et al (1995). In contrast restriction activity may decrease cortical representation of different muscles. Liepert et al (1995) have demonstrated a significant decrease in the cortical motor representation of inactive leg muscles after 4-6 weeks of unilateral ankle immobilisation and was more pronounced when the duration of immobilisation was longer. Investigation following amputation of part of upper limb revealed that the remaining muscles of that limb received more descending connection than the equivalent muscles of the intact limb (Hallet et al 1990).

Most striking is that following damaged or degenerated brain cells the functional representation may extent to the intact territories. Experiment carried out by Nudo et al (1996) have demonstrated that following a lesion to a small part of motor cortex that represent hand movement of the squirrel monkey, an intensive behavioural training of skilled hand use resulted in a prevention loss of hand territory adjacent to the infarct area. Moreover, this intensive training helped to expand the hand representations into region formerly occupied by representation of elbow and shoulder. It can be assumed that similar functional reorganisation of nerve cells may be facilitated in case degeneration of basal ganglia. Especially the function of the supplementary motor area, premotor cortex, and primary motor areas may be reorganised in order to compensate functional losses of basal ganglia. Moreover when PD subjects are exposed to challenging home activities, the impaired selective attention function, which is resulted from BG dysfunction, and which may be compensated by other aspects of attention like sustained or focused attention.

Conclusion

Human brain is endowed with a constant remodelling process depending on stimulation it receives. Task specific, goal directed activities helps to facilitate this changes. In contrast inactivity or a reduced activity may result in a stress deprivation of the brain, which may be responsible for the further deterioration of brain function.

There are two main types of changes in the brain have been identified, they are experience-depend change and functional reorganisation. Different experiences of learning and performing functions, which create a challenging environment, facilitate generation of new neuron as well as dendritic and axonal sprouting. Contrarily, experience deprivation a non-challenging passive living condition may not facilitate experience dependent change. Another type of change that can be expected in the brain is a functional reorganisation in the intact neural circuits in order to achieve the impaired functional goals in a different way. However, investigation on brain change is beyond the scope of this present research. Nevertheless this theoretical aspect needs consideration given the fact the designed movement strategies use the intact areas of the brain to generate movements, and therefore repeated use of different tasks may facilitate experience-dependent change and functional reorganisation in the intact neural circuits of the brain.

PD is the imbalance of neurotransmitter dopamine in the basal ganglia of the brain. The basal ganglia have widespread connection with different parts of the brain; therefore their dysfunctions produce a wide spread motor, cognitive and behaviour impairments. Among the motor dysfunctions akinesia or poverty of movement seems to be responsible for the progressive deterioration of functional activity level. Detailed movement analyses reveal that several underlying factors are responsible for the akinesia of movement, which include absence of automatic background movements, difficulty to initiate and execute movements, difficulty to perform large amplitude movement and finally extra difficulty to perform concurrent movements. Therefore if it is possible to counteract those difficulties it may help PD subjects to cope with the movement disorder which in turn may slow the disabling process. Counteracting akinesia will involve use an alternative strategy to perform functional activities that is use conscious voluntary movements, use visual and verbal cues, learn to prepare mental map every time before starting and activity, and finally learn to disintegrate simultaneous concurrent movements in to several simple acts. These alternative strategies presumably help PD subjects to generate movements using other intact motor areas of the brain by bypassing the defective BG. Moreover it may be expected that that repeated use of alternative strategy while performing functional tasks within the home environment may facilitate changes like experience-dependent change and functional reorganisation in the intact neural circuits of the brain. These changes in the intact neural circuits may result in a long-term improvement in functional activity level and slow the process of disability in PD subjects. However PD subject may have different types of cognitive impairment on the top of motor dysfunction and these cognitive dysfunctions may have adverse effect on relearning of motor function moreover they may be barrier for fostering change in the intact neural circuits. Therefore PD subjects with severe cognitive impairment will need special cognitive rehabilitation program and physical management alone may have very minimum impact on their activity level.

It seems that determining the most significant strategy to counteract different factors responsible for akinesia in PD subjects has the potential to improve functional activity level. However there is no research based evidence on the long term effect of alternative strategies on akinesia and on activity level in subjects with idiopathic PD. Therefore it seems relevant to conduct a clinical control trail to obtain more insights on the tasks difficulties in PD at home and the impact the movement strategies on functional status in PD subjects.

References

Abbruzzese G, Berardelli A (2003) Senseriomotor integration in movement disorders, Moveemnt disorder 18 : p231-240.

Afifi, A.K. (1993) Basal ganglia: functional anatomy and physiology. Part 2 [review]. Journal of child Neural; 9: P352 – 61.

Alexader GE, Dze Long MR, Strick PL. (1986) Parallel organisation of functionally segregated circuits linking basal ganglia and cotex. Annu. Rev. Neurosci. 9, 357 – 81.

Alexander GM and Crutcher MD (1990) Functional architecture od basal ganglia circuits: neural substrates of parallel processing. Trend of neurosci. 13: 266- 271.

Asanuma and Keller (1991) in Meara and Koller (2000) 'Parkinson's Disease and Parkinsonism in the Elderly. Cambridge University Press;, Cambridge, UK

Bach-y-Rita; P (1989) Theory based neurorehabilitation. Archive of Physical medicine and Rehabilitation; 70, 162.

Banks MA, and Caird FL (1989) Physiotherapy benifits patients with Parkinson disease. Clinical rehabilitation. 3, 11 – 16.

Behrman AL, Tietelbaum P, Cauraugh JH (1998) Verbal instructional sets to normalise the temporal and spatial gait variables in Parkinson's disease. Journal of Neurology, Neurosurgery and Psychatry. 65: P. 580-582.

Benecke et al (1986) in Morris ME, (2000) Movement Disorder in People with Parkinson Disease: A model for Physical Therapy. Physical Therapy. Volume 80. No 6. P578-597.

Benecke et al (1987) in Morris ME, (2000) Movement Disorder in People with Parkinson Disease: A model for Physical Therapy. Physical Therapy. Volume 80. No 6. P578-597.

Benecke R, Rothwell J C, Dick JPR, et al (1997) in Morris ME, (2000) Movement Disorder in People with Parkinson Disease: A model for Physical Therapy. Physical Therapy. Volume 80. No 6. P578-597.

Berardelli, A., Dick J.P.R. Day, B.L and Marsden, C.D. (1986) Scaling of the size of the first agonist EMG burst during rapid wrist movements in patients with Parkinson's disease. Journal of Neurology, Neurosurgery and Psychiatry 49: 1273-1279.

Bhatia KP and Marsden CD (1994), 'The behavior and motor consequences of focal lesion of the basl ganglia in man'. Brain 117(pt4): P 895-876.

Bleton, J.P. SteveninP.H. (1985) Rééducation dans le traitement de la maladie de Parkinson. Encycl. Méd. Chir. Paris, Kinésithérapie. 4-4-10.

Brotchie P, Iansek R, HornMK (1991) Motor function of monkey globus pallidus, neuranal discharge and parameter of movement. Brain, 114(pt4): 1667-1683.

Cameron, H.A.et al (1993) 'Differentiation of newly born neurons and ganlia in the dentate gyrus of the adult rat', Neuroscience 12, 3642-3650.

Can- J, Shepherd R. Neurological Rehabilitation: Optimizing Motor Performance. Oxford, United Kingdom: Butterworth-Heinemann; 1998.

Cao, J. Wenberg, K. Cheng, M.F. (2002) Lesion induced new neuron incorporation in the adult hypothalamus of the avian brain. Brain Research. 943; 80-92.

Carr J, Shepherd R (1998) Optimising Motor performance. Oxford, UK: Butterwort-Heinemann.

Carr J; and Shepherd R (2004) Stroke rehabilitation, guidelines for exercise and training to optimize motor skill. Elsevier Scientific Limited, London.

Chen YC et al (1995) in Meara and Koller (2000) 'Parkinson's Disease and Parkinsonism in the Elderly. Cambridge University Press;, Cambridge, UK.

Cools, R (2006), Dopaminergic modulation of cognitive function- implications for L-DOPA treatment in Parkinson's disease. Neuroscience & Behavioural Reviews; Volume 30, Issue, Page 1-53.

Cruz-Martinez A (1984) 'Electrophysiological study in hemiparatic subjects: electromyography, motor conduction and response to repetitive nerve stimulation'. Electroencephalogr. Clin Neurophysiol., Vol 20 P139-148.

Cunnington R, Iansek R, Bradsaw J, Phillips J H, (1995) Movement-related potential in potential in Parkinson disease: Presence and predictability of temporal and spatial cues. Brain. 118(pt 4):n 935-950.

Day, B.L, Dick, J.P.R and Marsden, C.D. (1984) Patients with Parkinson's disease can employ a predictive motor strategy. Journal of Neurology, Neurosurgery and Psychiatry. 47, 1299-1306.

De Goede CJ Kaus SH Kwakkel G, Wagenaar RC (2001) The effects of of physical therapy in Parkinson's disease: a research synthesis. Arch. Phys. Med. Rehabil.; 82: 509-515.

Denny-Brown D, and Yanagisawa N (1976) The role of basal ganglia in the initiation of movement. InYahr MD edition, The basal ganglia.Raven Pres, New York.

Denzin, N.K.and Lincoln, Y.S. (1994) Handbook of Qualitative Research, Sage, London.

DePoy & Gitlin (1998) Introduction to research understanding and applying multiple strategies Mosby, Inc.:120-122, 188-193, *Dietrich M. Brandt T (1992) in Carr J; and Shepherd R (2004) Stroke rehabilitation, guidelines for exercise and training to optimize motor skill. Elsevier Scientific Limited, London.

Dong Y, Dobkin BH, Cen SY, Wu AD, Winstein CJ. Motor cortex activation during treatment may predict therapeutic gains in paretic hand function after stroke. Stroke. 2006;37: 1552-1555.

Dong Y, Winstein CJ, Albistegui-DuBois R, Dobkin BH. Evolution of fMRI activation in the perilesional primary motor cortex and cerebellum with rehabilitation training-related motor gains after stroke: a pilot study. Neurorehabil Neural Repair. 2007;21:412-428.

Ellis T, De Goede J, Feldman RG, et al (2005) Efficacy of a Physical Therapy Program in Patients with Parkinson's Disease: A Randomized Controlled Trail.

Eriksson, P.S. et al (1998) Neurogenesis in the adult human hippocampus Nat.Med.4, 1313-1317.

Eriksson, P.S. et al (1998) Neurogenesis in the adult human hippocampus Nat.Med.4, 1313-1317.

Evarts, E.V. Teravainen, H. and Calne, D.D. (1981) 'Reaction time in Parkinson's disease.' Brain, 104: 167- 186.

Farmer S F, Swash M, Ingram DA et al (1993) Changes in motor unit synchronization following central nervous lesion in man. Journal of Physiology, Vol463, P 83-105.

Flowers K.A;, Robertso C, (1985) The effect of Parkinson's disease on the ability to maintain a mental set. Journal of Neurology, Neurosurgery and psychiatry, 43, 517-529.

Formisano R, Pratesi I Moderalli F Bonifati V, Meco G,(1992) 'Rehabilitation and Parkinson's disease.' Scand J Rehab Med 24, P157-160.

Fuster et al (1980) in Zomeren, Van, A.H. and Brouwer, W.H., (1994). Clinical Neuropsychology of Attention. NewYork: Oxford University Press.

Galletly R, and Braure S (2005) Does the type of concurrent task affect preferred and cued gait in people with Parkinson's disease? Australian Journal of Physiotherapy. 51: 175-180.

Georgiou et al (1993) in Meara and Koller (2000) 'Parkinson's Disease and Parkinsonism in the Elderly. Cambridge University Press;, Cambridge, UK.

Gibberd F, Page N, Spencer K, Kinnear E, Hawksworth J Hawksworth J, (1981) 'Controlled trial of physiotherapy and occupational therapy for Parkinson's disease.' BMJ, 282, 1196.

Goldberg G, (1985) Supplementary motor area: Structure and function: review and hypotheses. Brain and behavioural sciences. 36: 567 – 616.

Goldenberg G, Lang W, Podreka I, Deeecke L (1990) Are cognitive deficits in Parkinson's disease caused by frontal lobe dysfunction? Journal of psychology, 4, 137-144.

Goodrich S, Henderson L, Kennard C (1989) On the existence of an attention-demanding process peculiar simple reaction time: Converging evidence from Parkinson's disease Cognitive Neuropsychology, 66. 309-331.

Gould, E. et al (1997) 'Neurogenesis in the dentate gyrus of the adult tree shrew is regulated by psychological stress and NMDA receptor activation', Journal of Neuroscences.17. 2492-2498.

Gould, E., Tanapat, P., Hastings, N.B., Shors, T.J. (1999) Neurogenesis in adulthood: a possible in learning. Trend in Cognitive Sciences – Vol. 3. P. 186 – 192.

Greenfield J, Bosanquet F (1953) The brain-stem lesions in Parkinsonism. J Neurol Neurosurg Psychiatry.;16:213-226.

Guba, E.G. and Lincoln, Y.S. (1994) 'Competing paradigms in qualitative research'. In

Guyton, A.C. (1981) A text book of Medical Physiology. W.B. Sanders Company.

Heilman, M.K. Ven Den Abell, T. (1997) Right hemisphre dominancefor mediating cerebral activation. Neuropsychologia, 17, 315-321.

Higgs, J. Titchen A. (1998) 'Research and Knowledge' Physiotherapy, February, Vol. 84, no2.

Holden A, Wilman A, Wieler M, Martin W (2006) Basal ganglia activation in Parkinson's disease, Parkinsonism related disorder. 12:73-77.

Holden A, Wilman A, Wieler M, Martin W. Basal ganglia activation in Parkinson's disease. Parkinsonism Related Disord. 2006; 12:73-77

Holden A, Wilman A, Wieler M, Martin W. Basal ganglia activation in Parkinson's disease. Parkinsonism Related Disord. 2006;12:73-7

Hömerg, V. (1993) 'Motor training in the therapy of Parkinson's disease' S46 Neurology, 43 (suppl. 6) December.

Hughes AJ, Daniel SE, Blankson S, Lees AJ. (1993) 'A clinicopathologic study of 100 cases of Parkinson's disease'. Arch Neurol. 50:140-14.

Human Skill: A Multidisdplinary Approach. Champaign, 111: Human Kinetics Inc; 1998:329-354.

Huxham F. (2006) Turning During Gait in Parkinson's Disease [doctoral dissertation]. Melbourne, Victoria, Australia: La Trobe University.

Iansek R, Bradshaw J, Phillips J, et al (1995) Interaction of the basal ganglia and supplementary motor area in the elaboration of movements. In: Glencross D, Piek J, eds. Motor control and sensoriomotor integration. Amsterdam, The Netherlands : Elsevier; 37-59.

Jankovic J and Tosa H (1988) 'Parkinson's disease and Movement disorders'. Baltimore, Md: Urban and Schwarzenberg (eds).

Jankovic J, Nutt J G, Sudarsky L (2001) in Morris M. E. (2006) 'Locomoton Training in People with Parkinson's Disease'. Physical Therapy, Volume 86, Number 10, October

Jenkins et al (1990) in Carr J; Shepherd R (2004) Stroke rehabilitation, guidelines for exercise and training to optimize motor skill. Elsevier Scientific Limited, London.

Johansson BB (2000) in Carr J; Shepherd R (2004) Stroke rehabilitation, guidelines for exercise and training to optimize motor skill. Elsevier Scientific Limited, London.

*Jueptener M, Frith C, Brook D et al (1997) Subcortical structures and learning by trial and error. Journal of Neurophysiology. 77: 1325-1337.

Kampermann G, Kuhn H G, and Gage F h, (1998) Experence induced neurogenesis in the senescent dentate gyrus. Journal of Neurosciences 18, 3206-3212.

Kampermann, Brandon, E.P., Gage, F.H. (1998) Environmental stimulation of 129/Svj mice caused increased cell proliferation and neurogenesis in the adult dentate gyrus. Curr. Biol. 8, 939-942.

Kampermann, G. Kuhn, H.G., Gage, F.H. (1997) More hippocampal neurones in adult mice living in an enriched environment. Nature 386, 493-49.

Kandel E.R.; Schwartz J.H; Jessel T. M. (2000) Principals of Neural Science (Fourth edition) Mc Craw – Hill Companies, New York.

Kelly S W, Jahanshashi M, Dinberger G (2004) 'Learning of ambiguous versus hybrid sequences by patients with Parkinson's disease'. Neuropsychologia; 42, P1350-1357.

Kirkwood B. (1997) Occupational therapy for people with Parkinson's disease. In: Morris ME, Iansek R, eds. Parkinson's Disease: A Team Approach. Victoria, Australia: Biscombe Vicprint; 83-104.

Krefting L (1989) 'Reintegration in the community after head injury: the result of ethnographic study, Occup. Ther. J. Res. 9 P67-83.

Kuhn, T. (1970) The Structure of Scientific Revolution (2nd Edition), Chicago: University of Chicago Press.

Lewis S JG; Dove A; Robbins TW, Barker RJ; Owen AM; (2003) Cognitive Impairments in Early Parkinson's Disease Are Accompanied By Reduction in Activity in Frontostriatal Neural Circuitry. The Journal of Neuroscienc, July, 23(15 P6351 – 6356.

Liepert J et al (1995) in Carr J; Shepherd R (2004) Stroke rehabilitation, guidelines for exercise and training to optimize motor skill. Elsevier Scientific Limited, London.

Liston and Tallis (2000) in Meara and Koller (2000) 'Parkinson's Disease and Parkinsonism in the Elderly. Cambridge University Press;, Cambridge, UK

Luria (1973) The working brain. Penguin press, London.

Luria, A.L. et al. (1975) 'Restoration of higher cortical functions following local brain damage.' Handbook of clinical of clinical neurology (Vol. 3) (Vinken, P.J.and BrruynG.W. eds). Page 368-499.

Majsak MJ, Kaminski T, Gentile AM, Flanagan RJ, (1998) 'The reaching movements of patients with Parkinson's disease under self-determined maximal speed and visually cued conditions.' Brain121(pt 4), P755-766.

Mak M.K.Y, and Cole J.H, (1991) Movement dysfunction in patient with Parkinson's disease: A literature review; Australian Physiotherapy; Vol.37, no.1, 1991. 7-17.

Mak M.K.Y. and Hui-Chan (2008) 'Cued task-Specific Training is Better Than Exercise in Improving Sit-to-Stand in Patients with Parkinson's Disease: A randomised Controlled Trial.' Movement Dsorders

Marsden CD (1984); Which motor disorder in Parkinson's disease indicates the true motor function of basal ganglia? In Evert D and O'Connor M (eds), Function of the Basaal Ganglia. Ciba foundation Symposium 107/ London PitmanPublishing P. 225-241.

Marsden, C.D. (1989) 'Slowness of movement in Parkinson's disease', Movement Disorders, 4, 1, 26 – 36.

Marsden, CD (1982) The mysterious motor function of the basal ganglia. The Robert Wartenberg lecture. Neurology (NY), 32, 514 – 539.

Martin J P, (1967)' 'The Basal Ganglia and Posture'. London. Pitman Medical.

Meara and Koller (2000) 'Parkinson's Disease and Parkinsonism in the Elderly. Cambridge University Press;, Cambridge, UK.

Morris M E, (2005) Impairments, activity limitation and participation restriction in Parkinson's disease. In: Refshauge K, Ada L, Ellis eds. Science based Rehabilitation: Theories into practice. London, UK, Butterworth Heinemann ; 223-248.

Morris M E, and Iansek R (1997) Gait disorder in in Parkinson's disease : a framwark for physical therapy practice. Neurol. Rep. 21; P125-131

Morris M E, Iansek R, Matyas T A, Summers J J,(1995), 'Motor control considerations for gait rehabilitationin Parkinson's disease'. In: GleccrossD, Piek J, eds. Motor control and Sensorimotor Intigration. Amsterdam, the Netherlands: Elsevier, P 61-93.

Morris M. E. (2006) 'Locomoton Training in People with Parkinson's Disease'. Physical Therapy, Volume 86, Number 10, October

Morris ME, (2000) Movement Disorder in People with Parkinson Disease: A model for Physical Therapy. Physical Therapy. Volume 80. No 6. P578-597.

Morris ME, Collier J, Matyas TA, et al (1998) Evidence for motor skill learning in Parkinson's disease. In PiekJ. Ed Motor Behaviour and Human Skill: A multidisciplinary approach Champaign, III: Human Kinetics Inc, 329-354.

Morris ME, Collier J, Matyas TA, et al. Evidence for motor skill learning in Parkinson's disease. In: Piek J, ed. Motor Behavior and

Morris ME, Iansek R, Matyas TA, Suuers JJ, (1995), 'The Pathogenesis of gait hypokinesiain Parkinson's disease. Brain. 117 (pt5): 1169-1181.

Morris MF, Iansek R, Matyas TA, Summers JJ (1996). Stride length regulation in Parkinson's disease: normalization strategies and underlying mechanisms. Brain. 1996; 119 (pt 2): 551 – 568.

Neudo, R.J. et al (1996) Use-dependent alterations of movement representation in primary motor cortex of adult squirrel monkeys. Journal of Neurosciences. 16. 785 – 807.

Nieuwboer A, De WeerdtW, Dom R, Truyen M, Janssens L, Kamsma Y (2001) 'The effect of a home physiotherapy program for persons with Parkinson's disease'. Journal of Rehabilitation Medicine, 33, P 266-272.

Nudo et al (2001) in Carr J; Shepherd R (2004) Stroke rehabilitation, guidelines for exercise and training to optimize motor skill. Elsevier Scientific Limited, London.

Papa, S.M, Artieda, J. and Obeso, J.A. (1991) Cortical activity preceding self-initiated and externally triggered voluntary movements, Movement Disorders, 6,3, 217-224.

Pasual –Leone A, et al (1995) in Carr J; Shepherd R (2004) Stroke rehabilitation, guidelines for exercise and training to optimize motor skill. Elsevier Scientific Limited, London.

Pasual-Leone A, and Torres F (1993) in Carr J; Shepherd R (2004) Stroke rehabilitation, guidelines for exercise and training to optimize motor skill. Elsevier Scientific Limited, London.

Pasual-Leone A, Grafman J, Clarke K, Stewart M, Massaquoi S, Lou J S, Hallett M (1993) Procedural learning in Parkinson's disease and cerebellar degeneration'. Ann. Neurol., 34 P 594-602.

Polger S, Morris M E, Reilly S, Bilney B, Sanberg PR (2003) 'Reconstructive neurosurgery for Parkinson's disease: a systematic review and preliminary meta-analysis'. Brain Research Bulletin, 60. P 1 -24.

Rauch S, Whalen P, and Savage C, et al (1997) 'Striatal recruitment during and implicit sequiebce learning tasks as measurbed by functional magnetic resonance imaging'. Human Brain Mapp, 5 P124-132.

*Recanzone, G.H., Schreiner, C. E. and Merzeinch, M. M. (1993) Plasticity in the frequency representation of primary auditory cortex following Discrimination Training in Adult Owl Monkeys. The Journal of Neuroscience. 13(1). 87-103.

*Riggolati G. Camarada R. (1987) in Robertson. I.H. (1999) Cognitive rehabilitation: Attention and neglect. Trend in Cognitive Sciences – Vol. 3. No. 10.

Robertson. I.H. (1999) Cognitive rehabilitation: Attention and neglect. Trend in Cognitive Sciences – Vol. 3. No. 10.

Rochester L, Hetherington V, JonesD, et al (2004) 'Attending to the tasks: interference effects of functional tasks on walking in in Parkinson's disease and role of cognition, depression, fatigue and balance.' Achieve of Physical Medicine and Rehabilitation. 85, p1578-1585.

Scandalis T, Bosak A, Berlinger J, et al (2001) Resistance training and gait function in patients with Parkinson's disease', American Journal of Physical medicine and Rehabilitation, 80, P38-43.

Schenkman M, Cutson T M, Kuchibhata M, Chanler J, Piper C F, Ray L, Laub K C, (1998) 'Exercise to improve spinal flexibility and function for people with Parkinson's disease: a randomized controlled trial.' J. Am. Geratr. Soc 46: P 1207-1216.

Schmidt, R.A. (1982) Motor Control and learning. Illinos: Human Kinetic publishers.

Schultz W, Apilcella P, Romo R, Scarnati E (1995) 'Contex-dependent activity in primate striatum reflecting past and future behavioral events. In: Houk JC, Devis JL, Beiser DC, edsModels of information processing in the basal ganglia. Cambridge, Mass: The MIT Press; P11-27.

Seitz RJ, and Roland P, (1992) 'Learning of sequential finger movements in man: a combined kinematic positron emission tomography study.' European Journal of Neurosciences, 4: pp 199-207.

Selby G (1975) Parkinson disease. In: Vinken PJ. BruynGW, eds. Handbook of clinical neuropsycholog. 2nd ed, the Netherlands: Elsevier; 173-211.

Shumwau-Cook A, and Woollcott M (1995) 'Motor control: theory and practical applications'. Philadelphia: William and Wilkins

Sidaway B, Anderson J, Danielson G, et al. (2006) Effects of long-term gait training using visual cues in an individual with Parkinson disease. Phys Ther. 86:186–94.

Sinkjaer T Magnussen I. (1994) in Carr J; Shepherd R (2004) Stroke rehabilitation, guidelines for exercise and training to optimize motor skill. Elsevier Scientific Limited, London.

Smith E.E., JonidesJ, (1999) Storage and executive process in the frontal lobe, Science 283, PP1657-1661.

Spires TL, and Hannan AJ, (2005) Nature, nurture and neurology: gene-environment interaction in neurodegenerative disease. FEBS Journal. 272: 2347-2361.

Squire L R, Odo L R, Knowlton B, Musen G (1993) 'The structure and organisation of memory' Annual Review Psychology, 44, P453-495.

Talland G, Scwab R, (1964) 'Performance with multiple set in Parkinson's disease', Neurophysiologia. 2: P45-53.

Thaler et al (1995) in Meara and Koller (2000) 'Parkinson's Disease and Parkinsonism in the Elderly. Cambridge University Press;, Cambridge, UK.

TillersonJL, Cohen AD, Caudle WM, et al (2002) Forced nonuse in unilateral parkinsonian rats exacerbates injury. Journal of neurosciences. 22:6790-6799.

Van Veeramah (2002), On line Class, Lotus Note, Greenwich University.

Ward NS, Brown MM, Thompson AJ, Frackowiak RS. Neural correlates of outcome after stroke: a cross-sectional fMRI study. Brain. 2003;126:1430-1448.

Weissenborn S. (1993) The effect of using a two-step verbal cue to a visual target above eye levels on the parkinsonian gait: a case study. Physiotherapy, January 1993, vol.79, no.1.

Winter DA (1987) 'The Biomechanics and Motor Control of Human Gait, University of Waterloo Pres, Waterloo, Ontario.

Woodlee MT, SchallertT. (2004) The inteplay between behaviour and neurodegeneration in rate models in Parkinson's disease and stroke. Restor. Neurol. Neurosci; 22: 153-161.

Zomeren, Van, A.H. and Brouwer, W.H., (1994). Clinical Neuropsychology of Attention. NewYork: Oxford University Press.

REHABILITATION OF PEOPLE WITH TRAUMATIC PARAPLEGIA

I
Introduction

In traumatic paraplegia the damage in the spinal cord produces sensory and motor impairment below the level of lesion, along with urinary bladder, bowel and sexual dysfunction. The severity of impairment depends on the severity of cord lesion, weather complete or incomplete; and on the level of spinal injury. Immediate muscle and sensory impairment may follow secondary complications like bed sores or pressure sores, urinary tract infection and chest infection. Rehabilitation strategy is to teach patient how to cope with the disability inflicted due muscle and sensory impairment of the lower limbs and the lower part of the trunk. The following discussion briefly describes the strategies to prevent immediate complication like bed sore, and chest infection. Then the discussion highlights some of long-term managements, which include maintain range of motion of paralysed limbs and bladder management, wheelchair management, and finally the ability to live at home and in the society in a wheel chair.

II

Management in the Acute Stage, During Bed Rest Period

- Assure immobility of the fracture site
- Prevent pressure sore
- Prevent urinary tract infection
- Prevent chest infection
- Maintain length of soft tissues and prevent joint deformity.

Treatment in the initial stage (acute stage): Immediate after the spinal injury the main complication can arise as a result bed rest. However surgical intervention with internal fixation techniques has largely reduced the bed rest period and has minimise the complication rate. During bed rest period, the desensitised skin becomes highly susceptible to develop pressure sores. Therefore prevention of pressure sores is one of the main objectives of the treatment. Other complications include, urinary tract infection, chest infection, shortening of soft tissues and joint deformity.

Prevention of pressure sore: Desensitised skin following a spinal cord injury is become vulnerable to develop pressure sores. Pressure sore occurs due to prolonged pressure on the skin. The prolonged pressure on the skin is responsible for an avascular necrosis of the area under pressure. Depending on the duration of pressure the skin and underlying tissues will be affected. It is important to take into account that the skin subjected to two hours in a constant pressure can be enough to initiate necrosis of the tissues. The skin under the bony prominence like skin area over sacrum, trochanter, malleolus, are vulnerable to develop pressure sore. Given that the sore is the direct result of pressure, relieve of pressure is the best strategy to prevent pressure sore. The strategies to prevent pressure sore include special matress, change of position of the patient two hourly, cleanliness of skin and bed, watching of the skin regularly.

Special mattress: Special air mattress is available prevent pressure sore. In this mattress different parts of the bed is inflated and deflated in a regular basis in order to alleviate pressure from the skin, without interfering normal blood flow to the area.

Regular turning: In the absence of special mattress, regular turning of the patient is essential to prevent pressure sore. Each patient is moved from prone lying to right side lying, then to left side lying, and again to prone position. The turning needs to be continued every two hours during twenty four hours.

Cleanliness of the skin and the bed is also important to prevent pressure sore. Moisture of bed and the skin makes it venerable for skin breakdown. Therefore clean and dry skin is important in the prevention of bed sore.

Regular inspection of the skin areas susceptible to develop pressure sore: A regular inspection of the skin over bony prominences is essential to detect the initiation of pressure sore. As soon as any sign of pressure sore appears, even it is a minimum sign, immediate action need to be taken to prevent any further pressure on the area until the sign is completely subsided.

Prevent joint deformity: Prevention of joint deformity and the contracture of soft tissues of the paralysed limbs: During bed rest, the immobility in a non-weight bearing position may provoke atrophy of soft tissues and bones. The atrophy is mainly due to the deprivation of normal stress required for maintaining the strength, resilience and the thickness of the tissues. The atrophy of the tissues is followed by their contractures, giving rise to deformity of the joint and limb. Passive mobilisation and passive stretching of soft tissues help to prevent contracture of tissues and deformity of the joint to a certain extent. Despite the fact passive movement cannot provide the normal stress that is required to prevent stress deprivation, nevertheless it can prevent contracture and deformity of the tissues to a certain extent.

Urinary bladder management: Disturbance of bladder function produces many complications which constitute a life-long threat to the patient Bromley (1981). The main complication is urinary tract infection is common in people with paraplegia. Different management strategies exist to evacuate urine. People who use indwelling catheter for micturition are susceptible of getting urinary tract infection. Despite the extreme care of aseptic technique used to introduce catheter the rate of urinary tract infection is high. Therefore at the National Spinal Injury Centre, Stoke Mandeville Hospital, UK has developed intermittent catheterisation. Some people continue self catheterise after the acute phase is over. People with paraplegia especially with automatic or reflex bladder can evacuate their urinary bladder by manual pressure above the symphysis pubis. Different Spinal Injury Centres have adapted their own urinary bladder management strategy. (For a detailed information on Bladder management developed at the National Spinal Injury Centre, Stoke Mandeville Hospital, UK see, Bromley I (1981) Tetraplegia and Paraplegia: A Guide for Physiotherapists. Ed. Churchill Livingstone)

Prevention of chest infection: Capacity of respiratory function often reduces with the paralysis of abdominal muscles in many people with traumatic paraplegia. Moreover bed rest also slows respiratory function. Theses in turn can be responsible for the development of chest infection. It is therefore important take necessary measures to prevent chest infection especially in the early post-traumatic and post-operative stage. Chest infection prevention measure includes practice deep breathing exercise – which include diaphragmatic, lateral costal and apical breathing.

II

Treatment in the Chronic Stage When Bed Rest is Over

Once the fracture is consolidated or stabilised by internal fixation and paraplegic subject is allowed to sit the rehabilitation program of chronic stage starts. The rehabilitation program of complete paraplegia includes strengthening of upper limb and trunk muscles to be able adapt to live in a wheel chair; prevent deformity and contracture of joint and soft tissues of the paralysed limb; and finally learn to live by using a wheel chair.

Progressive standing practice:

As soon as fracture site is stabilised paraplegic patient is made standing with support progressively using tilt table. Both the duration of inclination and the degree of inclination have to be progressive in order to prevent the postural hypotension.

Improve sitting balance:

Good sitting balance is essential for paraplegic people for the management of wheel chair and to perform transfers to and from the wheel chair. Sitting balance is practice in a high sitting position on the edge of the plinth. At the beginning sitting with support using each hand on either side, then progress to sitting without support, and finally sitting without support and physiotherapist applies pressure to destabilise in different direction in order to improve stability in sitting position.

Strengthening of the upper limb and trunk muscles:

It is important to develop the muscles of upper limb and the trunk in order to be able to adapt living within a wheelchair. Different progressive strengthening exercises using pulley, weight can be used for strengthening upper limb muscles. Reinforcement of trunk muscle is also essential to maintain upright position.

Learn to use wheel chair in daily life activities:

Paraplegic people need to learn to be able to execute transfers to and from the chair safely. The transfer training can include, transfer from lying to sitting; transfer from bed to chair; transfer from wheel chair to chair, transfer to and from wheel chair to toilet sit; transfer from wheel chair to floor and from floor to wheel chair. It is also important to learn to transfer to and from wheel chair to car.

a) Laying ➔ Sitting; Sitting ➔ Laying.
b) Bed ➔ Wheel chair; Wheel chair ➔ bed
c) Wheel chair ➔ Chair; Chair ➔ Wheel chair
d) Wheel chair ➔ toilet commode; Toilet commode ➔ Wheel chair
e) Wheel chair ➔ floor; Floor ➔ Wheel chair
f) Wheel chair ➔ Car Car ➔ Wheel chair.

Reintegration into social, professional life and participate sportive activities:

Once paraplegic subject has learned to use wheel chair in daily life activities, the next step is to return home and to reintegrate in the socio-professional life. Paraplegic subject learn to perform passive movement of the joints and passive stretching of soft tissues lower limbs and continues at home in a regular basis. It is important to participate in sportive activity. Wheelchair sports are becoming more and more popular, and many paraplegic subjects can continue sportive activities along with their professional activities.

Conclusion: A fracture of the vertebra causes damage of the spinal cord. The damaged spinal cord is unable to convey nerve impulses to the periphery, which is responsible for muscle and sensory impairment. Impairment depends on the severity of the lesion and the level of the lesion. A partial damage causes partial paraplegia that is some of the sensory and motor function can be intact, whereas a complete damage of the spinal cord produces a complete paraplegia. The above discussion has highlighted rehabilitation strategies for a complete paraplegia, which include prevent complications in the initial stage, and then rehabilitation strategies in the chronic stage that is when paraplegic subject is allowed to sit and use a wheel chair. The prevention of complication in the initial stage includes, prevention of pressure sore, prevention of urinary tract infection, chest infection and maintain joint range of movement. The treatment strategy in the chronic stage includes wheel chair management, able to return home and able to use wheel chair at home. And finally reintegrate in socio-professional and practice some sportive activity.

Reference:

Bromley I. (1981) Tetraplegia and Paraplegia: A Guide for Physiotherapists. Ed Churchill and Livingstone, Edinbourg

PHYSICAL MANAGEMENT GUIDE FOR PEOPLE WITH MULTIPLE SCLEROSIS

Introduction

Multiple sclerosis (MS) is mostly a demyelisation of white matter however gray matter lesions that is neuronal cell bodies, dendrites can also be found. Demyelinised nerve fibres hinder the nerve conduction, which produces neurological impairment and the presence of damaged gray matter can aggravate different neurological symptoms. Therefore neurological impairments depend on the nerve fibres that are damaged, and the areas of gray matter that are affected. Given that the disseminated nature of lesion, MS can produce a wide range neural impairments, and therefore it can be characterised by a wide range of neurological symptoms, which can include motor, sensory, cognitive, and behavioural impairment. Physical intervention to restore motor function and uphold functional activity level can be achieved by providing appropriate planned intervention to restore impaired neuronal function. Restoration of motor function includes the restoration different structure of motor neuronal functional architecture. Moreover balance impairment is also a common feature in MS, therefore the restoration of balance function is also essential in order to attain functional autonomy. The following discussion briefly highlights the physiopathology of MS. Then the discussion explains some of the strategies to restore the impaired architectural structure that mediates motor activities. Balance impairment is one of the common neurological symptoms in MS therefore the discussion has also highlighted some of the intervention strategies to improve balance function. The aim of physical intervention is to maintain and improve activity level; therefore a brief discussion is made on the possibility of people with MS to improve activity level and be involved in aerobic activities, which eventually may slow the progression of disease process. People with MS may present a wide spread cognitive impairment, which can have hindering effect on facilitating neural plasticity, therefore a brief discussion has highlighted the cognitive impairment and the possibilities to facilitate neuronal changes in MS.

II

Physiopathology of MS

Multiple sclerosis (MS) is an inflammatory predominantly, but not exclusively, involving the normal-appearing white matter (Giancarlo Comi 2010). In about 85% of the people with MS, defined relapsing–remitting (RR) MS, the early phase of the disease, is marked by acute attacks characterised by unifocal (two-third of patients) or multifocal white matter lesion (Wingerchuk and Weinshenker 2000); gray matter lesions are not frequent in early phase of the disease (Giancarlo Comi (2010). Moreover Bangalore et al (2010, p29) suggests that MS is characterised by a highly variable pattern of disease progression with some patients displaying a relapsing –remitting course and others displaying a progressive course. Demyelisation also causes axon to become vulnerable to irreversible degeneration and may possibly trigger degeneration of their neuronal cell bodies, and thus set the stage of disease worsening (Banglore et al 2010, p29). They further suggest that as might be expected from lesion dissemination, MS is characterised by multiple neurological deficits. Neurological dysfunction resulting from conduction block is usually transitory; however, the possibility of persistent conduction block cannot be excluded (Giancarlo Comi 2010). On the other hand the functional consequences due to axonal loss are irreversible if not compensated by CNS plasticity and axonal regeneration which seems to be quite modest at the best (Giancarlo Comi 2010). Inflammation followed by demyelisation of nerve fibres, which interferes the propagation of conduction of action potential. This interference of neural transmission can cause different neural symptoms, depending on the areas demyelinised and the extent of demyelisation. Demyelinised axon is responsible for exude of acetylcholine out of axon before arriving at the neuromuscular junction, which in turn can exhaust the reserve of acetylcholine. This unavailability of acetylcholine at the neuromuscular junction can create an inability to produce muscle contraction and people with MS can experience extreme fatigue. In contrast an interposition of rest between activities may allow the restoration of acetylcholine reserve to restart new muscle activities. The fatigability of individual with MS and the time of rest required for the restoration of acetylcholine reserve are dependent on the extent of myelin damage. Therefore different exercises are done by interposing rest between each exercise, which again need to be adjusted according to physiopathological state of each individual. Motor deficit is one of the main symptoms which results from the interference and propagation of action potential. The interference of propagation of action potential can impair the functioning the architectural structure that mediates motor activities, which in turn disrupts the kinematic organisation of motor activities. Motor functional architecture has three distinct entities; in MS one or several structure of these entities can be impaired. Moreover sensory, cognitive and balance impairment are also prevalent in MS. Physical management of MS encompasses identifying the aspect which is degenerated the aspect that remain intact

III

Physical Management of Motor Impairment in Multiple Sclerosis

In multiple sclerosis the inflammation of myelin followed by their degeneration can produce a wide spread neurological symptoms depending on the area affected and the extent of the damage. The neurological symptoms that are prevalent in multiple sclerosis consist of impaired balance function, and impaired motor, sensory and cognitive function. People with Multiple sclerosis can present with one or several of those symptoms. Physical management strategies have to be organised in order to restore impaired neural function, with an objective to improve functional activity level and the quality of life of each individual. That is the strategy of physical management strategy needs to integrate the activities that can minimise clinical symptoms responsible for the functional impairment. Therefore the following discussion highlights separately the physical management strategies to restore some of the main functional impairment in MS.

Restore balance function

Possible strategies to restore balance function:

Balance dysfunction is one of the common symptoms present in people with multiple sclerosis. The ability to balance in an upright position whether it is in sitting or in standing involves a coordinated action of different neuromuscular activities. Balance function is not only essential to maintain upright position, but also it enables one to readjust with ongoing postural changes during different activities. Therefore impaired balance function can severely hinder the ability to perform different activities of daily living, which in turn may be responsible for the decline of activity level in MS subjects. Moreover different musculo-skeletal structure as well as different neuronal units may be subjected to a stress deprivation as a result of reduced activity level, which can lead to a further deterioration of activity level. Therefore the restoration of balance function is essential so that MS subject can effectively readjust with the ongoing postural changes during functional tasks, which in turn can help to uphold their level of activity.

Carr and Shepherd (2004) suggest that ongoing postural adjustment involves:
- Supporting body mass over the lower limb;
- Moving the body mass from one lower limb to the other or one position to another;
- Responding rapidly to any threat to balance.

Cerebeller ataxia and sensory ataxia are the two main symptoms that are prevalent in MS, and which constitute the underlying cause for the impaired balance function. Ataxia is uncoordinated movement of the limbs and the trunk. In cerebellar ataxia the function of the cerebellum is impaired, which produces uncoordinated movements, whereas in sensory ataxia the symptoms are produced due to impaired deep sensation.

Cerebellar ataxia:

The ongoing postural adjustment requires coordinated action of voluntary, involuntary and reflex muscle activities (program, feedback and reflex controlled muscle activities), as well as intact sensory and cognitive function. The coordinated muscle action is largely mediated by the cerebellum and its connections. Therefore the dysfunction of cerebellum can cause severe impairment of balance and muscle coordination. One of the features of movements produced by cerebellum is synergic movements, which is the coordinated contraction of agonist and antagonist muscles to produce a smooth, well-controlled movement Ghez and Fahn (1985). Ghez and Fahn (1985) further describe the following movement abnormalities in a lesion of cerebellum:

- Dysmetria, inaccurate range and direction, amplitude, and force, as well delays in the initiation of movement;
- Decomposition of movement, in which the various the various components of an act are not executed in a smooth sequence;
- Hypermetria is an excessive extent of movement, as when a limb overshoots the desired point;
- Hypometria is a deficient extent of movement so that the limb stops before reaching the goal;
- Dysdiadochokinesia, and irregular pattern of alternating movements.

The above movement dysfunctions are identified as the cerebeller ataxia. Cerebellum not only produces coordinated movements but also maintaining upright position and adapt with constantly changing environment are mediated by cerebellum. Therefore people with cerebeller dysfunction experience difficulty to maintain upright position and to respond rapidly to any threat to balance in upright position. Consequently they compensate by increasing the double leg stance phase of walking slowing the pace of walking as well as widening the base of double leg stance. According to Ghez and Fahn (1985), cerebellum with their connections with vestibular system functions in maintaining upright position. Vestibular apparatus of internal ear contains sensory receptor which provides sensation of upright position of the body. Moreover some of the above symptoms can also present in people with impaired deep sensation, which falls in the category of sensory ataxia. In sensory ataxia, the symptoms can be minimized using visual control during activities; in contrast in case of cerebellar lesion the visual control unable to produce any change in uncoordinated movements. In multiple sclerosis the prevalence balance dysfunction can be either a sensory ataxia or cerebellar ataxia, in rare case both sensory and cerbellar ataxia can be present.

Specific intervention for the cerebellar ataxia:

Learning of progressive positioning, which consists of maintaining the most stable position then progressively learn to maintain the least stable position. Waddington (1989) suggests that in order to improve stability and minimise cerebellar ataxia the therapist can decide to apply rhythmic stabilization technique. A gradual increase of alternative resistance is used to build up co-contraction. Rhythmic stabilisation is effective to improve static stability, that is, the stability is improved in a static position. Therefore transfers from bed to chair, or chair to chair can be practiced with security once static sitting balance is achieved. Similarly walking with security can only be assured once static standing is achieved. Once the static stability is achieved the dynamic activities can be practice from that position. Repeated transfers from bed to chair, chair to bed, to start with under supervision, and then without supervision can improve sitting balance. Walking with support, under supervision, then without supervision, progress to waling without support and finally without support and without supervision can be practiced to improve dynamic stability in standing. Moreover resisted walking, where therapist apply resistance against walking forward as well as lateral walking, can also be practiced to improve dynamic stability in standing.

Sensory ataxia: In sensory ataxia uncoordinated movements are produced due to impaired deep sensory function. In sensory ataxia the sensory information regarding the position of the and limb and the joint does not reach up to the higher centre, which in turn produces the similar symptoms as cerebral ataxia. The symptoms of sensory ataxia can be minimized using visual sensation, whereas the symptoms in cerebral ataxia remains unchanged even the movements are done under the visual control. Therefore the use of visual sensation, which helps to minimise the dysmetria or hypermetria of movements that occur due to impaired deep sensation, can be effective.

Restore the structure of motor functional architecture:

Myelin degeneration in MS blocks the propagation of nerve impulse to facilitate muscle activities; moreover gray matter degeneration may also be responsible for the fewer neurons available for producing muscle activities. This in turn is responsible for the breakdown of architectural structure of the central nervous system that mediates motor activities. Therefore the restoration of functional architecture is essential to uphold functional activity level in people with MS. The objective of physical intervention is to facilitate neuroplasticity at level of gray matter, and to maximise the capacity of intact nerve fibres.

Restoration of program control system:

Program control system produces previously learned muscle activities. These activities are usually stored in the brain as a whole program and can be retrieved to achieve desired goal. Unlike in hemiplegic people in MS the programmed activity of individual or multiple limbs can be affected. The demyelinised neurons can interrupt the link between program control system of the brain with the periphery. Not only the programmed activity of one or multiple limbs may not be available, but also their reflex activities may be deprived of the modulating and inhibiting effects. Restoration of programmed control system is therefore essential, which can effectively exert its modulating and inhibiting effects on the reflex controlled activities. Strategies to restore program controlled activities include; – improve individual muscle function, – improve the whole chain of muscle activities, – and finally learning functional tasks. A detailed discussion has highlighted the strategies to restore program control system on the chapter on stroke rehabilitation.

Restore feedback control system

Feedback control system generates individual muscle activities. Sensory function and voluntary effort play essential role in generating feedback controlled activities. People with MS may have difficulty to generate feedback controlled activities due to the demyelisation of neuron as well as degeneration of nerve fibres. Feedback control system produces individual muscle activities. Impaired feedback control system produces weakness and loss of dexterity of individual muscles. The weakness and loss of dexterity of individual muscle may fail to exert inhibiting and modulating effect on reflex activities of muscles, producing muscle spasticity. Therefore increase strength and dexterity of individual muscle can help to restore program control system and effectively minimise uninhibited reflex activities of the muscles.

Management of spasticity:

As discussed in the previous chapter that spasticity is involuntary muscle contraction results from an uninhibited reflex activity of muscle and posture. Spasticity is characterised by increased muscle tone and abnormal limb movement. Uninhibited postural reflex is more prevalent in post-stroke hemiplegic and in cerebral palsy; in contrast in case of multiple sclerosis spasticity is mainly due to uninhibited muscle reflex and postural reflex hyperactivity is less frequent. The normal reflex muscle activities are deprived of the inhibiting and modulating effects of feedback and program controlled muscle activities, causing uninhibited reflex activities or spasticity. Given that the spasticity has resulted from impaired program controlled and feedback controlled muscle activities, therefore the restoration of these two systems constitutes an essential strategy to minimise spasticity. Some of the strategies minimise spastic pattern of the limb are already discussed in the treatment of hemiplegic people.

IV
Improve Functional Activities Level and Engaging in an Aerobic Activity

Given that the plastic changes in the neuronal tissues are facilitated by active repeated and task-specific activities, therefore the objective motor sensory and balance re-education is to improve functional activity level in people with MS. The improved activity level not only helps to facilitate plastic changes in the neural tissues, but also helps to uphold structure and function of different contractile and non-contractile tissues of the limb and trunk, due to the fact that they are practice repeatedly throughout the day and every day.

Engaging in an aerobic activity:

Different aerobic activities not only strengthen the structure of musculoskeletal structure but also help to improve the structure of neural tissues. In contrast a minimised activity level may accelerate the degenerative process of neural tissues, which can make them vulnerable to a new relapse of the disease process. Moreover different aerobic activities may help to minimise depression and anxiety related to a reduced activity level. Most clinicians acknowledge that psychological factors have a profound effect on the outcome of treatment in people suffering from chronic condition (Maly et al 2005). Rudy et al (2005). Aerobic exercises, like walking program, running, aquatic exercises, yoga, and Tai Chi have been shown to be effective in improving the functional status, gait, aerobic capacity in healthy people and people with chronic condition.

Moreover aerobic activities or an increased activity level may have positive impact on the self efficacy for physical tasks. Self-efficacy refers to a person's belief in his or her capability to organize and execute the actions required to achieve a wide range of goals (Bandura 1998). According to Lorig et al (1989) self-efficacy is the confidence that people have in their ability to perform a specific task. Self-efficacy may help people with MS to minimise the dominating role of the disease process on their life. Aerobic activities in MS have to be designed according the capacity of individual, the progression of disease process, and most important is that it has to be dosed while respecting the state of fatigue of each individual. Outdoor activities have to be avoided in case of extreme heat and cold.

V
Cognitive Impairment and Possibility to Facilitate Neural Changes in Multiple Sclerosis

People with multiple sclerosis may have wide spread cognitive dysfunctions, which is dependent on the neural areas that are affected. Different cognitive impairments can have a hindering effect in the process of relearning of movements and reacquisition of functional autonomy. Common cognitive dysfunctions in MS include attention, memory, and executive dysfunction. More detailed discussion is made on different cognitive dysfunction, their repercussion of motor learning process, as well as some of the strategies to overcome their hindering effects in the chapter on rehabilitation of post-stroke hemiplegic subjects.

Possibility to facilitate neural change in multiple sclerosis:

Like any other neurological conditions, plastic changes in the neural cells can be facilitated in people with MS. These plastic changes or neuronal regeneration include experience dependent-change, functional reorganisation, and lesion induce neuronal proliferative activities. Active, repeated and task-specific activities are effective for the facilitation of neuroplasticity. In contrast inactivity or reduced activity may fail to facilitate the process of neuronal regeneration. Different cognitive impairment can have hindering effect on neuronal regeneration. Given that MS is an autoimmune attack to myelin sheaths and oligodendrocytes, and the activities to facilitate plastic changes of neuronal tissues may have very little effect on myelin regeneration. However some evidence has recently accumulated to indicate that an axonal and synaptic pathology could accompany or even precede the central nervous system autoimmune infiltration (Vercellino et al 2005, Dutta and Trapp 2007, Chard and Miller 2007). Moreover Zimarino et al (2010) state that in people with chronic MS, together with standard white matter lesions seen by brain imagining techniques, some degree of cortical and deep gray matter lesion have been found, and since gray matter is composed of neuronal cell bodies, dendrites, and synapses, these findings indicate an alteration of one more of these neural structures. It can be assumed that different neuronal plasticity can be facilitated within these structures. Zimarino et al (2010) suggests that the progression of neuropathological damage initiated by the removal of myelin sheaths which alternatively might also derive from compensatory or plastic changes at the level of either upstream or downstream neuronal structure. However active and repeated task-specific activities and precisely shaped therapeutic intervention facilitate compensatory plastic changes. In contrast inactivity and the absence of therapeutic intervention may fail to facilitate plastic changes. Therefore the precisely shaped therapeutic intervention and tasks specific-activities, when they are practiced in a repeated manner, can help not only to hinder the deterioration of gray matter neuronal structures but also can facilitate their regenerative process.

VI

Conclusion

Multiple sclerosis (MS) is mostly a demyelisation of white matter however gray matter lesions that is neuronal cell bodies and dendrites can also be found. Demyelisation is mainly due to an inflammatory degeneration of myelin sheath. Deprived of their myelin sheath the nerve fivers are unable to conduct neuronal impulses. This is mainly because the acetylcholine, which is an essential neurotransmitter, is unable to propagate within the nerve fibres. Given that the disseminated nature of lesion of MS, it can produce a wide range of symptoms, depending on the area affected and the severity of lesion. The symptoms of MS include motor, sensory, cognitive, and behavioural. Physical intervention strategy includes uphold level of functional and aerobic activity. The strategy to improve of motor function includes restoration of functional architecture responsible for the kinematic organisation of motor activities. Many people with MS can have impaired balance function; therefore it is essential to undertake strategies to improve balance function. Moreover people with MS can have wide range of cognitive impairment and impaired cognitive function can have hindering effect on facilitation of neuronal plasticity. Different précised activities to restore impaired neural function may not be able to facilitate regeneration of myelin; however those activities can strengthen the undamaged nerve fibres. Moreover different neuronal plasticity can be facilitated at the level of impaired gray matter.

References:

Kesselring J., Gaincarlo C Thompsoson A.J., (2010) Multiple Sclerosis: Recovery of Function and Neurorehabilitation, Ed. Cambridge University press, UK.

Gaincarlo C (2010) in Kesselring J., Gaincarlo C Thompsoson A.J., (2010) Multiple Sclerosis: Recovery of Function and Neurorehabilitation, ed. Cambridge University press, UK.

Wingerchuk D.M., and weinshenker B.G. (2000) in Kesselring J., Gaincarlo C Thompsoson A.J., (2010) Multiple Sclerosis: Recovery of Function and Neurorehabilitation, ed. Cambridge University press, UK.

Bangalore L. Black J.A., Carrithers M.D., Waxman S.G., (2010) in Kesselring J., Gaincarlo C Thompsoson A.J., (2010) Multiple Sclerosis: Recovery of Function and Neurorehabilitation, ed. Cambridge University press, UK.

Carr J; and Shepherd R (2004) Stroke rehabilitation, guidelines for exercise and training to optimize motor skill. Elsevier Scientific Limited, London.

Kandel E.R., Schwartz J.H. (1985) Princiciples of Neuroral Science, 2nd edition, Elsevier Science Publishing CO. Inc, New York.

Ghez C. And Fahn S (1985) in Kandel E.R., Schwartz J.H. (1985) Princiciples of Neuroral Science, 2nd edition, Elsevier Science Publishing CO. Inc, New York.

Maly M.R., Costitigan A., Olney S.R. (2005) 'Contribution to psychological and mechanical variables to physical performance measures in knee osteoarthritis'. Physical Therapy, Vol. 85 p1318-1324.

Rudy e., Zhang W. Dorothy M., (2005), 'Aerobic walking or strengthening exercise for osteoarthritic knee?' A systematic review. Am. Rheu. Dis64, p196-202.

Bandura E. (1998) 'Health promotion from perspective of socio cognitive theory'. Psychol. Health, 13 p623-649.

Lorig K. Gongalez V. Laurent D. et al (1989) in Maly M.R., Costitigan A., Olney S.R. (2005) 'Contribution to psychological and mechanical variables to physical performance measures in knee osteoarthritis'. Physical Therapy, Vol. 85 p1318-1324.

Vercellino M ; Plano F. Votta B. et al (2005) in Kesselring J., Gaincarlo C Thompsoson A.J., (2010) Multiple Sclerosis: Recovery of Function and Neurorehabilitation, Ed. Cambridge University press, UK.

Dutta R., and Trapp B.d. (2007) in Kesselring J., Gaincarlo C Thompsoson A.J., (2010) Multiple Sclerosis: Recovery of Function and Neurorehabilitation, Ed. Cambridge University press, UK.

Chard D. and Miller D. (2007) in Kesselring J., Gaincarlo C Thompsoson A.J., (2010) Multiple Sclerosis: Recovery of Function and Neurorehabilitation, Ed. Cambridge University press, UK.

Zimarino V. Ripamonti M. Belfior M, FerroM. Malgaroli A. (2010) in Kesselring J., Gaincarlo C Thompsoson A.J., (2010) Multiple Sclerosis: Recovery of Function and Neurorehabilitation, Ed. Cambridge University press, UK.

www.ingramcontent.com/pod-product-compliance
Lightning Source LLC
Chambersburg PA
CBHW020728180526
45163CB00001B/156